The Canadian
Clinician's
Rheumatology
Handbook

Second edition

Edited by
Lori Albert, MD

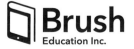

Brush
Education Inc.

Brush Education Inc.
www.brusheducation.ca
contact@brusheducation.ca

Cover design: Dean Pickup; Cover image © Tallik, Dreamstime.com
Interior design: Carol Dragich, Dragich Design
Editorial: Barbara A. Every
Illustrations: Chao Yu

Image credits: Hannah M. Yaphe and Elan Yaphe: Figures 19.1, 19.2,
19.3, 19.4; Dr. Nigil Haroon, Figure 19.6.

Library and Archives Canada Cataloguing in Publication
The Canadian clinician's rheumatology handbook / edited by Lori
Albert, MD.

Revision of: Canadian residents' rheumatology handbook /
edited by Lori Albert; Post-Graduate Education Working Group,
Canadian Rheumatology Association. — 1st ed. — Victoria, B.C. :
Trafford, 2005.

Includes bibliographical references and index.
Issued in print and electronic formats.
ISBN 978-1-55059-604-5 (pbk.).—ISBN 978-1-55059-605-2 (pdf).—
ISBN 978-1-55059-606-9 (mobi).—ISBN 978-1-55059-607-6 (epub)

1. Rheumatology—Handbooks, manuals, etc. I. Albert, Lori,
1963–, author, editor II. Title. III. Title: Rheumatology
handbook.

RC927.C26 2015   616.7'23   C2014-908483-8
                                          C2014-908484-6

We acknowledge the financial support of the Government of Canada
through the Canada Book Fund for our publishing activities.

Canadian   Patrimoine
Heritage   canadien

Dedication

To JY, H, and E

Table of Contents

Preface

The first edition of the *Canadian Clinician's Rheumatology Handbook* was entitled the *Canadian Residents' Rheumatology Handbook*, and it was designed to enhance and support a national rheumatology curriculum for core internal medicine trainees in Canada. Over the years, the book has been a helpful resource to medical students, family physicians, allied health professionals, and others. Thus, this second edition is more broadly geared to all Canadian clinicians, both trainees and those in practice, to help provide a starting point in the approach to common presenting problems of patients with rheumatologic disease.

Introduction

The *Canadian Clinician's Rheumatology Handbook* is designed to give the clinician a starting point in assessing the patient who presents with a particular rheumatologic syndrome. The *Handbook* provides a foundational approach and will help guide the user to identify where further reading in a standard textbook or current literature will optimize care of the patient. Chapters on the use of laboratory investigations and imaging provide a quick reference to enhance the ordering and interpretation of these tests. The "Selected Rheumatologic Emergencies" section will help the clinician to quickly get organized in the face of an acutely ill patient and will lay the groundwork for appropriate investigation and management. Finally, the sections on physical examination and joint injection techniques will serve as a refresher for some clinicians or as an introduction for others. Joint injection techniques, however, cannot simply be learned from a book, and the clinician should endeavor to have supervised practice before routinely doing these procedures. It is impossible to list every reference and additional resource in a small space, but many chapter authors have tried to provide some key references for further reading. Several excellent standard rheumatology textbooks can provide a structured and detailed approach to build on the learning in this book. Management of rheumatic diseases is a rapidly evolving area—searching the current literature is the best approach when more detail is required.

We hope that you enjoy using the *Canadian Clinician's Rheumatology Handbook* and anticipate that it will enhance your comfort and proficiency with the approach to the presenting problems of patients with rheumatologic disorders.

Lori Albert
September 2014

SECTION 1: APPROACH TO COMMON PRESENTATIONS OF RHEUMATIC DISEASES

Monoarthritis

DR. DOUG SMITH
UNIVERSITY OF OTTAWA

KEY CONCEPTS

Pain and swelling of a single joint (monoarthritis) often develops acutely. Understanding the differential diagnosis allows for a targeted history and physical examination that can help narrow the diagnostic possibilities. If trauma is excluded as a cause, the diagnosis will, in most cases, fall into 1 of 3 groups of conditions:

- **Infections:** It is most important to diagnose and treat infections quickly!

- **Crystals:** This group includes gout or pseudogout.

- **Seronegative spondylarthritis (SpA) (peripheral SpA):** This group includes reactive arthritis, psoriatic arthritis, and enteropathic arthritis.

Consider the following key steps in developing the differential diagnosis:

1. Determine if there is a history of trauma.
2. Decide if the process is articular or nonarticular.
3. Use clues from the history and physical examination to narrow the differential diagnosis (age, gender, risk factors, previous episodes, family history, back pain, travel history). The presence of extra-articular manifestations is particularly helpful.
4. Obtain laboratory data. These data may be supportive, but generally cannot be used to make the diagnosis in isolation.

5. Aspirate the joint and analyze synovial fluid to firmly establish the diagnosis and guide therapy.

History

PATIENT DEMOGRAPHICS

Any age: Think infectious causes.

Young men and women: Think infection (especially *Neisseria gonorrhea*) and SpA. Remember, young women do not get gout!

Older men and women: In the absence of infection (higher risk in elderly patients), crystal arthritis is likely.

KEY QUESTIONS

These questions seek to establish whether the patient has:

- a history of trauma
- previous episodes of acute joint inflammation
- a clearly articular process (versus a nonarticular or periarticular process)
- a history of risk factors for infection (e.g., travel, sexual activity)
- axial (spinal) involvement
- extra-articular features that can provide clues

1. Is there a history of trauma?

- An acute injury to a joint such as the knee may lead to hemarthrosis, particularly if there is a meniscal and/or cruciate tear.
- Trauma may also play a role in periarticular conditions such as olecranon or prepatellar bursitis.

2. Is this the first episode of acute joint inflammation?

Recurrent episodes are more suggestive of crystals or SpA.

3. Is this truly an articular process or is it nonarticular or periarticular?

- Periarticular inflammation may be confused with septic arthritis.
- In olecranon bursitis, the inflammatory process begins in the bursa and may extend to the soft tissues around the elbow. Extension of the knee is relatively preserved—unlike in an acute inflammation of the joint itself, where extension is lost early.
- In prepatellar bursitis, the inflammatory process begins in the bursa in front of the patella and extends to the soft tissues around the knee. Extension of the knee is relatively preserved—unlike in an acute inflammation of the joint itself, where extension is lost early.
- Periarticular inflammation of the ankles, when combined with erythema nodosum, is suggestive of acute sarcoidosis.
- Marked periarticular inflammation ("pseudocellulitis") can occur with gout and can mimic infection.
- Intense periarthritis can result from acute deposition of calcium hydroxyapatite crystals (classically in the shoulder, hip, and first MTP joint in young women, but can occur in other areas).

4. How did it come on?
- **Gradual and insidious onset:**
  - is typical for early onset of inflammatory arthritis such as psoriatic arthritis

- can be seen in septic arthritis in elderly or immunocompromised patients

- **Acute onset:**
  - is typical for infection or crystals
  - is also typical of reactive arthritis with a history of time lag after a precipitating GI or GU infection

5. Which joints are involved?

- **Septic arthritis** is most commonly due to the hematogenous spread of organisms from a site of primary infection. Joints affected tend to be medium to large, and are often weight-bearing joints, particularly those that have been previously damaged.

- **Gout** tends to involve the first MTP joint, the ankle, and the knee. In older women, it may affect the DIP joints of the hands with tophi superimposed on Heberden nodes (osteoarthritis).

- **Pseudogout**, which is due to calcium pyrophosphate dihydrate (CPPD) crystal deposition, commonly presents as an acute monoarthritis affecting a knee or wrist in older individuals.

- **SpA** (see chapters 2 and 8) can present with asymmetrical involvement of the lower extremities and the larger joints (knees, ankles).
  - There may be enthesitis (inflammation of the insertion of tendon and ligament into bone) at the Achilles tendon and at the plantar fascia insertion with heel pain.
  - There may be dactylitis (inflammation of the tendon sheath plus periostitis, producing "sausage digit") in patients with psoriatic arthritis and reactive arthritis.
  - The presence of inflammatory axial involvement also suggests SpA (see chapter 8).

Monoarthritis

6. Is there a history of travel, risk factors for sexually transmitted diseases, or other infections?

- Inquire about unprotected sex, multiple partners, and recent GU symptoms.

- Ask about IV drug use.

- In older individuals especially, a history of recent respiratory or GU infection raises concern for septic arthritis.

- Travel, especially to Lyme-endemic areas (see sidebar) may be relevant.

- See also chapter 13.

7. Are there any constitutional symptoms?

Fever suggests infection but is also seen with other causes, particularly crystals.

8. Are there any symptoms outside of the joints (extra-articular features)?

- Extra-articular features of SpA include the following: oral ulcers, conjunctivitis, uveitis, GU symptoms, GI symptoms, psoriatic rash, keratoderma blenorrhagicum, circinate balanitis, enthesitis, and dactylitis.

- Acute diarrheal illness preceding presentation of arthritis by 1 to 3 weeks suggests reactive (postdysenteric) arthritis.

- Urethritis/cervicitis, pustular skin lesions, and tenosynovitis may be present with disseminated gonococcal infection (may precede development of septic monoarthritis).

- Erythema migrans of Lyme disease appears and then disappears weeks or months before development of monoarthritis (see sidebar).

- The presence of tophaceous deposits (patient may report new lumps or bumps) supports a diagnosis of gout.

LYME DISEASE

Lyme disease is a tick-borne zoonosis caused by *Borrelia burgdorferi* and transmitted most commonly by the blacklegged tick, *Ixodes scapularis*.

This tick species is endemic to the northeastern United States, the Great Lakes region, the midwestern United States, and the western United States, including northern California and Oregon. It is also present in Canada and Europe.

In Canada, vector ticks sometimes infected with *B. burgdorferi* are reported in many provinces, but are found in 2 localized regions in particular: along the north shore of Lake Erie in Ontario (Point Pelee National Park, Rondeau Provincial Park) and in British Columbia in the Fraser delta, the Gulf Islands, and Vancouver Island, where the vector is *Ixodes pacificus*.

Lyme disease usually begins with a characteristic skin lesion (erythema migrans) and nonspecific symptoms such as fever, malaise, fatigue, headache, myalgias, and arthralgias. Erythema migrans is typically a small erythematous papule or macule that appears at the site of the tick bite after 1 to 2 weeks. The lesion subsequently enlarges with or without the development of central vesicles, necrosis, or a bull's-eye appearance.

Early dissemination may result in multiple erythema migrans lesions and manifestations affecting the nervous system (lymphocytic meningitis; cranial neuropathy, especially of the facial nerve and radiculoneuritis), the musculoskeletal system (migratory joint and muscle pain), and the heart (rare transient atrioventricular block).

Late disseminated disease (weeks to months after infection) most commonly manifests as intermittent arthritis of 1 or a few large joints, particularly the knee. About 10% of untreated patients develop chronic arthritis. Late neurologic manifestations include chronic axonal polyneuropathy and chronic encephalomyelitis.

9. Are there other medical illnesses?

- Inflammatory bowel disease could indicate enteropathic arthritis.
- Psoriasis could indicate psoriatic arthritis.
- Iritis or uveitis could indicate SpA.

- A history of diabetes, cirrhosis, immunosuppression, rheumatoid arthritis (RA), or HIV increases likelihood of an infectious cause.
- A prosthetic joint increases the likelihood of an infectious cause.
- Chronic kidney disease could indicate gout.
- Transplant patients could have gout (cyclosporine-related) or septic arthritis (immunosuppression).

10. What is the family history?

Seronegative arthritis, psoriasis, or inflammatory bowel disease in family members increases suspicion for first presentation of SpA.

11. What medications are currently being taken? What medications have been tried?

- Ask about medications the patient has tried and the response (e.g., anti-inflammatories, antibiotics).
- Ask about medications used for other reasons, for example:
  - Gout is exacerbated by diuretic use, low-dose ASA, and cyclosporine.
  - Immunosuppressive agents increase the risk for infection.
  - Anticoagulants may provoke hemarthrosis.

12. Have there been any previous investigations?

Have any blood tests, imaging studies, or synovial analyses been done previously that might give clues?

13. What is the social history?

Ask about:

- alcohol use, IV drugs
- sexual history, contacts
- risks for trauma

Physical Examination

Vital signs: Look for fever, tachycardia (signs of possible sepsis).

Head and neck: Look for ocular inflammation (think SpA), oral ulcers (painless with reactive arthritis, painful with enteropathic arthritis).

Chest: Examine the chest as a possible source of disseminated infection. Listen for crackles (apical fibrosis with spondylarthritis). Examine chest expansion as part of spine examination.

Cardiac exam: Listen for murmurs (consider bacterial endocarditis, aortic insufficiency with long-standing aortic stenosis).

Skin and nails:

Check for:

- psoriasis, nail pitting, onycholysis (think psoriatic arthritis)
- pustular skin lesions (think disseminated gonococcal infection)
- nodules (think tophi and gout)
- lesions on palms and soles (think pustular psoriasis and keratoderma of reactive arthritis)
- lesions on glans penis (think circinate balanitis of reactive arthritis)
- erythema nodosum (think enteropathic arthritis, acute sarcoidosis)

Neurologic exam: Check for encephalopathy. Note that neuropathy may present with late Lyme disease.

Musculoskeletal exam:

- Check for signs of inflammation such as erythema, warmth, or swelling or effusion (expected in monoarthritis).

- Note that acutely inflamed joints usually have limited range of movement.
- Check for swelling confined by the joint capsule (e.g., in the elbow: swelling due to an effusion is most apparent in the area between the olecranon process and the lateral epicondyle and does not extend over the olecranon process).
- Check for loss of extension (e.g., in the knee: significant effusion produces swelling and distention of the suprapatellar pouch, but generally does not extend anterior to the patella, thus causing loss of extension).
- Check for periarticular inflammation (e.g., olecranon bursitis, prepatellar bursitis), evident because of localization of swelling at the olecranon/patella, with preservation of joint extension, and painful and/or limited flexion.
- Look for additional sites of joint involvement (the patient may be unaware of these).
- Assess for spine involvement, particularly in young to middle-aged individuals (see chapter 8). However, findings on spine examination may be normal even in the presence of early evolving spondylarthritis.

Key Laboratory Investigations

BLOOD WORK

CBC: Look for leukocytosis and left shift as evidence of infection (not sensitive or specific).

ESR, CRP: These are not specific, but may support a more systemic inflammatory process if elevated.

Creatinine, urinalysis, liver function tests: Use as screening before therapy. Abnormal urinalysis could indicate evolving systemic disorder.

Serum urate: This is **not** helpful during an acute attack. Up to one-third of patients with acute gout have normal uric acid levels during acute attacks (the mechanisms are not entirely clear). A fall in uric acid (e.g., due to use of uric-acid-lowering medications) may have precipitated an acute attack.

Cultures of blood, urine, synovial fluid, etc: Use these to rule out infection. For gonococcal infection, include swabs of urethra, cervix, anus, and oropharynx.

JOINT ASPIRATION AND SYNOVIAL FLUID ANALYSIS

Note that the only significant contraindication to joint aspiration is evidence of infection in the needle path superficial to the joint (e.g., cellulitis or potentially septic bursitis, in which case aspiration should be of the bursa and not the underlying joint). Patients with monoarthritis affecting a prosthetic joint should be referred immediately to orthopedics.

Appearance: Fluid may appear clear (noninflammatory), turbid (inflammatory), purulent (infectious), or bloody (hemarthrosis or possible traumatic aspiration).

Cell count: A differential can distinguish normal, noninflammatory, and inflammatory monoarthritis. See Table 1.1. These are guidelines only!

Gram stain: Culture and sensitivity testing should also be done.

Crystals (see also chapter 10)

Urate: These are long, thin, needle-shaped crystals, which may be free in fluid and/or phagocytosed by

TABLE 1.1. Typical features of synovial fluid analysis in various causes of monoarthritis

	Normal	Noninflammatory (e.g., osteoarthritis)	Inflammatory (e.g., RA, crystals, SpA)	Septic
Appearance	Clear	Clear	Yellow, turbid	Opaque
Viscosity	High	High	Low	Low
Total WBCs $\times 10^6$/L	< 200	200–2000	2000–75 000	> 50 000*
% PMNs	< 25	< 50	> 50	> 75

Abbreviations: PMNs, polymorphonuclear leukocytes; RA, rheumatoid arthritis; SpA, spondylarthritis.

*Note that these are guidelines only. It is possible to have septic arthritis with cell counts < 50 000 $\times 10^6$/L.

WBCs (may appear to be pierced through). The crystals polarize brightly when visualized under a polarizing microscope, with strongly negative birefringence.

- If a crystal is aligned parallel to λ of the red compensator—usually indicated on the handle of the red compensator—the crystal appears yellow (**mnemonic**: parallel yellow).

- If a crystal is aligned perpendicular to λ of the red compensator, it appears blue.

Pyrophosphate: These are much smaller, broader, rhomboid-shaped crystals, and may be in fluid and/or phagocytosed inside WBCs. They polarize weakly (less brightly) and are positively birefringent—i.e., if a crystal is aligned parallel to λ of the red compensator, it appears blue; if it is perpendicular to λ, it appears yellow.

Pleomorphic crystals: Traces of injected steroid preparations appear as tiny pleomorphic crystals, which polarize brightly with intense negative or positive birefringence. Transient postinjection "flares" may be related to these crystals.

Note: Gout and septic arthritis may coexist!

ADDITIONAL TESTS

- Screen for Lyme disease only if the clinical picture is consistent and there is a history of travel to an endemic area, a known tick bite, or a history of erythema migrans rash.

- Enzyme-linked immunosorbent assay plus Western blot demonstration of antibody response to *B. burgdorferi* are interpreted according to Centers for Disease Control and Prevention guidelines. (**Note:** After 1 month of disease, most patients have positive IgG responses. For acute disease of less than 1 month, sensitivity of serological testing is low and should include both acute and convalescent serum samples.)

- Ascertain HLA-B27 status if SpA is suspected.

Imaging

PLAIN RADIOGRAPHS

- Use these for comparison of affected and contralateral joint.

- Plain radiographs are often insensitive and nonspecific, but may be helpful with chondrocalcinosis, if osteomyelitis is a concern or if a possible septic process is subacute. They may also reveal unsuspected fracture, osteonecrosis, or adjacent bone tumour as possible causes of monoarticular pain.

- In the setting of acute calcific periarthritis (due to hydroxyapatite crystals), amorphous calcific deposits may be seen in the tendons around the affected joints and are diagnostic. A classic example is acute periarthritis of the shoulder, with amorphous radiodense deposits in the supraspinatus tendon.

- Consider plain radiographs for SI joints and the lumbar spine if SpA is suspected.

Differential Diagnosis

There is a wide differential diagnosis for the patient presenting with monoarticular pain or inflammation. In the acute setting, the differential diagnosis can be organized according to the same categories outlined in "Key Concepts": trauma, infection, crystals, and SpA (Table 1.2). For chronic monoarthritis, the infectious organisms are different, crystal arthritis is restricted to gout, and

TABLE 1.2. Selected causes of acute monoarthritis

Cause	Outcome or agent
Infection	Bacteria: *Staphylococcus aureus* (most common overall)
	Hemolytic strep, gram-negative organisms (elderly, immunocompromised, chronic disease), *Haemophilus influenzae* (children)
	Neisseria gonorrhea
	Bacterial endocarditis
	Mycobacteria
	(See chapter 13)
Crystals	Gout
	Pseudogout (CPPD crystal deposition)
	Hydroxyapatite (acute calcific arthritis and/or periarthritis)
Traumatic	Hemarthrosis
Spondylarthritis (peripheral or axial)	Psoriatic arthritis
	Reactive arthritis (post chlamydia, post dysenteric)
	Ankylosing spondylitis (hip, sometimes knee)
	Enteropathic arthritis
Other	Hemarthrosis (secondary bleeding disorder), anticoagulation
	Palindromic rheumatism
	Sarcoidosis

Abbreviation: CPPD, calcium pyrophosphate dihydrate.

TABLE 1.3. Selected causes of subacute or chronic monoarthritis

Cause	Outcome or agent
Infection	Mycobacteria
	Fungi
	Lyme disease
	Bacterial
Inflammatory	Spondyloarthropathies: psoriatic, reactive, enteropathic, and ankylosing spondylitis (hip, sometimes knee)
	Seropositive disease (RA): occasionally first presentation
	Chronic gouty arthropathy
	Foreign body synovitis
Noninflammatory	Osteoarthritis with secondary inflammatory flare
	Hemarthrosis
Tumour	Pigmented villonodular synovitis
"Idiopathic"	Not evident, by definition (diagnosis may become evident over time)

Abbreviation: RA, rheumatoid arthritis.

chronic inflammatory arthritis (SpA or even RA) becomes more likely (Table 1.3).

Initial Therapy

Decisions regarding initial therapy for monoarthritis are made in the context of a complete history and physical examination, and the results of initial investigations as outlined earlier, including findings for synovial fluid appearance, cell count and differential, crystals, and Gram stain. Note that cultures of appropriate fluids will not be back in time to help with the initial treatment decision, but should be done at presentation.

Patients with monoarthritis affecting a prosthetic joint should be referred immediately to orthopedics for a decision regarding joint aspiration.

NONPHARMACOLOGIC THERAPY

- Rest, splinting, and ice packs may help reduce pain.

- Physiotherapy should begin when the acute situation is beginning to settle.

THERAPY FOR SPECIFIC PROBLEMS

Hemarthrosis

- Hemarthrosis secondary to trauma may be associated with a potentially significant internal derangement. An orthopedics referral is usually appropriate.
- Hemarthrosis secondary to an anticoagulation or clotting disorder may benefit from glucocorticoid injection to reduce the inflammatory response, if infection has been ruled out.

Suspected infection (see chapter 13)

- Antibiotic choices will depend on the suspected organism (gonococcal versus nongonococcal, gram-positive versus gram-negative), Gram stain, and local institutional recommendations.
- Consider involving orthopedics early with nongonococcal infection.

Suspected or proven crystalline arthritis

Options include the following:

- **Nonsteroidal anti-inflammatory drugs (NSAIDs):** If there is no contraindication, give the full dose of an NSAID for 10 to 14 days.
- **Oral glucocorticoids:** For example, give prednisone 20–40 mg in complicated cases where medical patients have underlying renal, hepatic, or cardiac disease.
- **Colchicine:** If the attack began less than 24 hours prior to presentation (ideally within a few hours), administer a 1.2 mg loading dose followed by 0.6 mg 1 hour later (avoid in patients with renal or hepatic disease). This can be followed by 0.6 mg once or twice daily until resolution.

- **Intra-articular steroid injection:** Consider this for an accessible joint if infection has been ruled out (see chapter 19).
- Do **not** start or stop urate-lowering drugs (e.g., allopurinol) during an acute attack, as this may worsen or prolong it.

Suspected SpA

- If there is no contraindication, give the full dose of an NSAID for 2 to 3 weeks and reevaluate.
- An intra-articular steroid injection can be used if infection is ruled out.
- Systemic glucocorticoids are considered only in patients with severe disease and in whom NSAIDs are contraindicated.

Further Reading

Khanna D, Khanna PP, Fitzgerald JD, et al; American College of Rheumatology. 2012 American College of Rheumatology guidelines for management of gout. Part 2: Therapy and antiinflammatory prophylaxis of acute gouty arthritis. *Arthritis Care Res (Hoboken)*. 2012;64(10):1447–61. http://dx.doi.org/10.1002/acr.21773. Medline:23024029

Shapiro ED. Clinical practice. Lyme disease. *N Engl J Med*. 2014;370(18):1724–31. http://dx.doi.org/10.1056/NEJMcp1314325. Medline:24785207

Monoarthritis

2

Polyarthritis and Polyarthralgia

DR. LORI ALBERT
UNIVERSITY OF TORONTO

KEY CONCEPTS

In the patient presenting with a polyarticular condition, the diagnosis may not be evident at the outset.

Some important features in the history and physical examination can help narrow the differential diagnosis early on. The diagnosis may also become clearer over time as the condition evolves.

The following key concepts should be considered in developing the differential diagnosis:

1. Decide if the process is inflammatory or noninflammatory.

2. Use clues from the history and physical examination to narrow the differential diagnosis (acuity, age, gender, joint distribution, and symmetry). The presence of extra-articular manifestations is particularly helpful.

3. Order focused investigations guided by clinical information. These laboratory data may be supportive, but generally cannot be used to make the diagnosis in isolation.

4. Follow the patient over time to firmly establish the diagnosis and refine therapy.

History

PATIENT DEMOGRAPHICS

Young men: Think viral and other infectious causes; reactive, psoriatic, enteropathic, or sarcoid arthritis.

Young women: Think viral and infectious causes, systemic lupus erythematosus (SLE), and rheumatoid arthritis (RA).

Older men: Think polyarticular gout (this usually coincides with a history of gout). Consider RA, psoriatic arthritis with appropriate history, and osteoarthritis.

Older women: RA is still likely. Consider polyarticular gout, as elderly women may present with involvement of smaller joints of the fingers. Consider calcium pyrophosphate dihydrate (CPPD) crystal deposition disease and osteoarthritis.

KEY QUESTIONS

These questions seek to establish whether the patient's condition:

- is acute or chronic
- is truly an articular process (versus nonarticular— e.g., polymyalgia rheumatica—or periarticular)
- is inflammatory or noninflammatory
- has a pattern of onset and a pattern of joint involvement
- has axial (spinal) involvement
- has extra-articular features that provide clues

1. How long have the joints been involved?
- If less than 6 weeks, the condition may be infectious (usually viral).

- Joint symptoms can also be the first presentation of chronic arthropathy.

2. Are there inflammatory features?
- Look for joint swelling (versus generalized soft tissue swelling or edema).
- Erythema implies more intense inflammation, and is typically seen only with infectious or crystal arthritis.
- Prolonged **morning stiffness** (more than 30 minutes to 1 hour) implies an inflammatory process.
- Look for decreased range of motion of affected joints and impaired function.

3. How did the condition come on?
- **Gradual and insidious onset:**
    - is typical for early onset of inflammatory arthritis such as RA or psoriatic arthritis

- **Acute onset:**
    - is typical for viral arthritis
    - is typical for reactive arthritis with history of 1- to 3-week time lag after a precipitating GI or GU infection
    - can be seen with RA, but less common (occasionally an explosive onset)

See Table 2.1 for patterns of polyarticular joint involvement that may provide a clue to diagnosis.

4. Which joints are involved?
- **Seropositive arthritis (typical pattern):**
    - is symmetrical
    - involves the small and large joints
        - MCP/PIP joint involvement with sparing of DIP joints
        - MTP involvement (common)
    - affects the upper and lower extremities

TABLE 2.1. Patterns of polyarticular Joint Involvement

Pattern of progression	Disease
Migratory – symptoms present in some joints for a few days, then remit, but new joints become involved	Infectious (*Neisseria* infections, rheumatic fever)
Additive – symptoms present in some joints and persist, and then new joints become involved and persist	Seropositive, some seronegative
Intermittent – attacks of multiple joint involvement with complete resolution between attacks	Crystal induced (polyarticular gout), early RA, palindromic arthritis, early psoriatic arthritis, reactive arthritis

Abbreviation: RA, rheumatoid arthritis.

- involves the spine **only** at the cervical level
- is the typical pattern seen in patients with seropositive connective tissue diseases such as systemic lupus erythematosus, scleroderma, myositis, etc., who have arthritis as part of their clinical picture

- **Seronegative arthritis associated with inflammatory spondylarthritis (SpA) (typical pattern):**
  - is asymmetrical
  - involves the lower extremities and larger joints with a predominately oligoarticular pattern
  - can have several possible patterns of joint involvement
    - Patterns unique to psoriatic arthritis include: an "RA-like" pattern; isolated DIP joint involvement (typically associated with nail changes of psoriasis); an oligoarticular pattern; a destructive, small joint "mutilans" pattern; axial involvement in combination with any of the other patterns.

- **Seronegative arthritis with axial involvement, enthesitis, or dactylitis:**
  - Axial spine involvement is the main manifestation in ankylosing spondylitis, but

may accompany peripheral joint disease in the setting of psoriatic arthritis, enteropathic arthritis, and reactive arthritis (see also chapter 8). The presence of inflammatory axial involvement is characterized by:

  o insidious onset
  o low back/buttock pain (often alternating buttock pain)
  o prolonged morning stiffness
  o waking in the second half of the night
  o pain relieved by activity

- Enthesitis is inflammation of the insertion of tendon and ligament into bone. Achilles enthesitis and plantar fasciitis are causes of "heel pain" in SpA.
- Dactylitis is inflammation of the tendon sheath—with or without synovitis, and with or without periostitis—producing "sausage digit." It is typically seen with psoriatic arthritis or reactive arthritis.

5. Are there any symptoms outside of the joints (i.e., extra-articular features)?

- Systemic disorders may present with fever, fatigue, and weight loss, which may suggest more significant inflammatory disease.
- Specific extra-articular features are most easily categorized according to seropositive and seronegative patterns (see Table 2.2).
- Extra-articular manifestations can also include:
  - tophi (gout)
  - erythema nodosum (sarcoidosis)
  - palpable purpura (small vessel vasculitis)
  - infection-related skin findings (hemorrhagic papules or vesicles, pustules of disseminated gonococcal infection, viral exanthems, etc.)
  - other manifestations

TABLE 2.2. Patterns of extra-articular manifestations

	Diseases	Extra-articular features
Seropositive	RA, SLE, other connective tissue diseases	Facial rash, other rash, photosensitivity, oral ulcers, alopecia, Raynaud phenomenon, sicca (dry eyes, dry mouth), serositis, nodules, pulmonary involvement
Seronegative	Reactive arthritis, psoriatic arthritis, enteropathic arthritis, ankylosing spondylitis, undifferentiated SpA	Oral ulcers, conjunctivitis, uveitis, GU symptoms, GI symptoms, psoriatic rash, keratoderma blenorrhagicum, balanitis, enthesitis, dactylitis

Abbreviations: RA, rheumatoid arthritis; SLE, systemic lupus erythematosus; SpA, spondylarthritis.

Polyarthritis

6. Are there any other medical conditions?
Inquire about:

- inflammatory bowel disease (enteropathic arthritis)
- psoriasis (psoriatic arthritis)
- iritis or uveitis (seronegative HLA-B27-associated diseases); other eye involvement (possible in RA)
- thyroid disease, diabetes, chronic kidney disease, etc. (musculoskeletal complaints—see chapter 7)
- recent symptoms of infection:
  - GU (reactive arthritis)
  - GI (reactive arthritis)
  - sore throat (rheumatic fever, viral infection)
    - Note that sore throat can also be a symptom of SLE, which is noninfectious.

7. Is there a family history of rheumatic diseases or related conditions?
Check for:

- SpA, psoriasis, inflammatory bowel disease
- RA or SLE (or other seropositive conditions)
- osteoarthritis

8. Are any medications being taken or has anything been tried to relieve symptoms?

- It is informative to learn which medications have been tried that help reduce symptoms (e.g., anti-inflammatories).

- Medications used for other reasons, especially new medications, may give clues to iatrogenic disease (e.g., drug-induced lupus, serum sickness reaction to penicillins, gout exacerbated by diuretic use).

9. What investigations, if any, have been done to date?

What, if any, blood work or imaging studies have been done that might give clues?

10. How do the joint symptoms affect functional capacity? How does the condition affect the patient's life?

Ask about:

- personal care: dressing, bathing, grooming, toileting
- daily activities: cooking, cleaning, shopping
- driving
- work and hobbies
- exercise, walking
- sexual function

This information can help guide the urgency and intensity of therapy.

Physical Examination

The goals of the physical examination are to identify the presence of inflammatory synovitis, to determine the pattern of joint involvement, and to look for clues that can point to a particular diagnosis. Rarely, patients presenting with polyarthritis are acutely ill, indicating the need for rapid assessment and management of an underlying inflammatory or infectious disorder.

Vital signs: Look for signs of systemic process or involvement of organs other than the joints: tachycardia, tachypnea, fever, hypertension.

Head and neck: Look for alopecia, ocular inflammation, oral and nasal ulcerations, nasal discharge or bleeding, malar rash, telangiectasia, lymphadenopathy, thyroid enlargement/nodules. Note that nasal discharge or bleeding may signal antineutrophil cytoplasmic antibody–positive (ANCA-positive) small vessel vasculitis.

Chest: Examine for tachypnea, crackles (interstitial lung involvement is associated with some rheumatic diseases), pleural effusions (SLE or RA). Examine chest expansion as part of spine examination.

Cardiovascular exam: Listen for murmurs (rheumatic fever, endocarditis), rubs (SLE, RA).

Skin and nails: Look for psoriasis or other rashes (SLE), periungual erythema (SLE and other connective tissue diseases), livedo reticularis (SLE with antiphospholipid antibody syndrome, vasculitis), nodules (RA), ulcerations (scleroderma, vasculitis), erythema nodosum (enteropathic arthritis, sarcoid), telangiectasia (limited scleroderma, mixed connective tissue disease).

Neurological exam: Examine for neuropathy (vasculitis, seropositive disease), carpal tunnel syndrome (possible with inflammatory arthritis involving the wrist), CNS abnormalities (SLE).

Musculoskeletal exam:

- Determine whether the involved joints show features of inflammatory synovitis or noninflammatory change (see also chapters 17 and 18).

- Active or inflamed joints are characterized on examination by joint-line tenderness or stress pain (pain with stressing just beyond the normal range of motion), warmth, erythema, effusion, and reduced range of motion.
- Damaged joints are characterized by joint-line tenderness, crepitus with movement, and reduced range of motion. Occasionally, small bland effusions may be present.
- Look for additional sites of joint involvement (the patient may be unaware of these).
- Assess for spine involvement (see chapter 8).
- Try to diagram the distribution of peripheral joints involved to look for a pattern. Figure 2.1 shows typical patterns of joint involvement for a variety of polyarticular conditions.

Key Laboratory Investigations

CBC: Look for anemia and thrombocytosis as signs of inflammation, cytopenias as part of a lupus picture, and lymphopenia secondary to viral infection or SLE.

Creatinine, urinalysis: Screen prior to therapy; look for signs of glomerulonephritis (SLE, vasculitis).

Liver enzymes:

- Screen prior to therapy; look for signs of hepatitis-related process.
- AST and ALT also arise from skeletal muscle and elevations may be a clue to an associated myositis.

ESR, CRP: There are not specific, but may support a diagnosis of a more systemic inflammatory process.

Special:

- Consider rheumatoid factor, anti-cyclic citrullinated peptide, antinuclear antibody, C3,

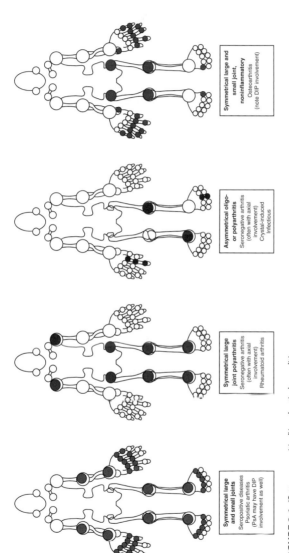

FIGURE 2.1. "Pattern recognition" in polyarticular conditions.

Symmetrical large and small joints
Seropositive diseases
Psoriatic arthritis
(PsA may have DIP involvement as well)

Symmetrical large joint polyarthritis
Seronegative arthritis
(often with axial involvement)
Rheumatoid arthritis

Asymmetrical oligo- or polyarthritis
Seronegative arthritis
(often with axial involvement)
Crystal-induced
Infectious

Symmetrical large and small joint, noninflammatory
Osteoarthritis
(note DIP involvement)

C4, ANCA, and HLA-B27 on the basis of clinical picture and pattern of arthritis (see chapter 10).

- Measure serum urate if clinical picture is suggestive of chronic polyarticular gout.

Imaging
See also chapter 11.

Plain radiographs:
- These are unlikely to be helpful with an acute process (radiographic changes within joints, such as erosions, are unlikely to be apparent until disease has been present for some time).
- In early stages of disease, plain radiographs may reveal soft tissue swelling, periarticular osteopenia.
- With more long-standing processes:
  - Consider X-rays of hands and feet (these can pick up early erosions in MTP joints, wrists, MCP joints).
  - Consider X rays of SI joints and lumbar spine if seronegative disease (SpA) is suspected.

Ultrasound with power Doppler: This may show changes of synovitis and early erosions (RA). It is not used routinely for this purpose, but may be helpful in specific cases.

MRI: This may show synovitis and early erosions (RA). It is not used routinely for this purpose, but may be helpful in specific cases.

Technetium bone scan: Consider this if you have difficulty in establishing a diagnosis (i.e., articular versus nonarticular).

Differential Diagnoses
The differential diagnosis to be considered depends on the duration of the symptoms. Within the first

6 weeks, infections, especially viral, can be the cause of polyarthritis, and close observation may be needed to see if arthritis persists over time (Table 2.3). If the polyarthritis has been present for more than 6 weeks, a chronic, persistent cause (i.e., autoimmune disease) is more likely (Table 2.4). Osteoarthritis is the most common

TABLE 2.3. Causes of acute inflammatory polyarthritis (less than 6 weeks)

Infectious	Noninfectious
Viral (rubella, hepatitis B and C, parvovirus, EBV, HIV)	Rheumatoid arthritis (new onset)
Bacterial (gonococcal, meningococcal)	Psoriatic arthritis
Bacterial endocarditis	SLE and other connective tissue diseases
Lyme disease (early)	Reactive arthritis
Acute rheumatic fever	Systemic vasculitis
	Polyarticular gout
	Serum sickness
	Sarcoid arthritis
	Palindromic rheumatism
	Still disease
	Familial Mediterranean fever
	Malignancy-associated arthritis

Abbreviations: EBV, Epstein-Barr virus; SLE, systemic lupus erythematosus.

TABLE 2.4. Causes of chronic polyarthritis (more than 6 weeks)

Rheumatoid arthritis

Psoriatic arthritis

SLE

Other connective tissue diseases

Reactive arthritis

Enteropathic arthritis or other seronegative arthritis (SpA)

Polyarticular gout

Still disease

Sarcoid arthritis

Malignancy-associated arthritis

Abbreviations: SLE, systemic lupus erythematosus; SpA, spondylarthritis.

Polyarthritis

TABLE 2.5. Causes of noninflammatory polyarticular symptoms

Osteoarthritis

CPPD crystal deposition disease

Metabolic/endocrine conditions (see chapter 7)

Others: hemochromatosis, ochronosis, acromegaly, benign hypermobility syndrome, hypertrophic pulmonary osteoarthropathy, hemophilia, sickle cell disease, amyloidosis, leukemia

Abbreviation: CPPD, calcium pyrophosphate dihydrate.

TABLE 2.6. Nonarticular causes of polyarticular pain

Polymyalgia rheumatica (primarily proximal pain and stiffness)

Fibromyalgia (pain, fatigue, and sleep disturbance)

Polymyositis (primarily weakness, occasionally pain)

Neuropathic pain

chronic noninflammatory arthropathy (Table 2.5). Nonarticular disorders can mimic polyarthritis and polyarthralgia, and should also be considered in the differential diagnosis (Table 2.6).

Initial Therapy

NONPHARMACOLOGIC THERAPY
Although every new patient with inflammatory polyarthritis may not need to see allied health professionals or may not have the resources to see them, treatment must include basic principles from these disciplines.

Occupational therapy
- Rest the affected joints.
  - Splints can be very effective for hand and wrist involvement.
  - Bed rest may be needed for extensive joint involvement.
- Use energy conservation principles (use periods of rest to maintain function).

- Use adaptive/assistive devices to minimize work of involved joints.

Physical therapy
- Ice acutely inflamed joints.
- Heat (e.g., hot wax) may be good for more chronically inflamed joints or osteoarthritis.
- Gentle exercise is needed early to prevent loss of function.
- **Patient education** is crucial to maximize adherence to investigations and therapy, and to maximize self-efficacy.

PHARMACOLOGIC THERAPY
See also chapter 12.

Nonsteroidal anti-inflammatory drugs (NSAIDs)
- Avoid NSAIDs if there is any suggestion of renal or hepatic involvement, or history of peptic ulcer disease.
- NSAIDs are the mainstay of initial management in many cases.
- NSAID choice depends on physician and patient preference, cost, availability, etc. Ensure therapeutic dose; monitor creatinine and liver enzymes.

Glucocorticoids
- These are appropriate for systemic rheumatic disease where diagnosis has been made or investigations are pending, infection has been ruled out, and NSAIDs are contraindicated or ineffective. Use the lowest dose possible.
- Sample doses:
  - **Polyarticular gout:** prednisone 25–30 mg/d for several days, then taper
  - **SLE:** prednisone 10–20 mg/d in absence of

other significant systemic disease; prednisone 0.5–1 mg/kg/d if there is internal organ involvement

- **Systemic vasculitis:** prednisone 1 mg/kg/d (with internal organ involvement)
- **Rheumatoid arthritis:** prednisone 10 mg/d or less—only recommended as a bridge while waiting for disease-modifying antirheumatic drugs (DMARDs) to work or if DMARDs are incompletely effective

- Oral single or divided dosing is usually acceptable as the route of administration.
- IV equivalents can be used in severely ill patients (see chapter 12).

Intra-articular glucocorticoids

Use these for individual, severely affected joints. Ensure infection has been ruled out.

DMARDs and immunosuppressive agents

- For chronic inflammatory polyarthritis (e.g., RA, psoriatic arthritis), DMARDs should be started early, as soon as diagnosis is confirmed, to minimize joint damage and reduce long-term sequelae. Therapy with these agents will also be required for patients whose arthritis is part of a systemic inflammatory disease that requires treatment.
- Consultation with a rheumatologist is recommended if these drugs are to be used.

Further Reading

Bykerk VP, Akhavan P, Hazlewood GS, et al; Canadian Rheumatology Association. Canadian Rheumatology Association recommendations for pharmacological management of rheumatoid arthritis with traditional and biologic disease-modifying antirheumatic drugs. *J Rheumatol*. 2012;39(8):1559–82. http://dx.doi.org/10.3899/jrheum.110207. Medline:21921096

Wevers-de Boer KV, Heimans L, Huizinga TW, et al. Drug therapy in undifferentiated arthritis: a systematic literature review. *Ann Rheum Dis*. 2013;72(9):1436–44. http://dx.doi.org/10.1136/annrheumdis-2012-203165. Medline:23744979

3

Muscle Weakness

DR. AURORE FIFI-MAH
UNIVERSITY OF CALGARY

KEY CONCEPTS

1. Weakness may reflect neuromuscular disease, in which case there is often an objective pattern of true motor impairment.

   - Patients will describe specific tasks that cannot be performed.

   - In evaluating the patient, consider pathology at the level of the muscle, the neuromuscular junction, the peripheral nerves, the spinal cord, and the central motor area.

2. Weakness can be a functional complaint, in which case there is no evidence of true weakness on examination.

3. A careful history and physical examination will help to distinguish the source of the patient's weakness. The distribution of muscle weakness (generalized versus localized, proximal versus distal, etc.) can be a helpful clue.

4. Inflammatory myositis—polymyositis (PM) and dermatomyositis (DM)—is characterized by progressive proximal muscle weakness and is the most common rheumatologic cause for muscle weakness.

5. Muscle weakness associated with muscle pain is rare and may indicate an underlying vasculitis.

6. Acute and severe generalized muscle weakness may reflect rhabdomyolysis and constitutes a medical emergency.

History

OVERVIEW

- The most common rheumatologic cause of muscle weakness is 1 of the idiopathic inflammatory myopathies.
  - PM is characterized by proximal, usually painless, muscle weakness that evolves insidiously over weeks to several months.
  - Commonly, the neck and shoulder girdle are involved first, and then the trunk and pelvic girdle.
  - Distal strength is usually not a major concern.
  - Dysphagia may be present, along with nasal regurgitation and aspiration.
  - Some patients may have associated interstitial lung disease.
  - Characteristic skin rashes suggest a diagnosis of DM rather than PM.
  - Inclusion body myositis, also an idiopathic inflammatory myopathy, is a less common disorder. It is more insidious in onset, seen in older individuals, may involve the lower extremities first, and can produce distal as well as proximal weakness.

- Many conditions can mimic PM/DM. Therefore, the history and physical examination must be directed toward confirming the classic features of PM/DM and ruling out neurologic, metabolic, or toxic/drug-related causes of muscle weakness.
- Distal symmetric or asymmetric muscle weakness that is associated with neurologic symptoms such

as paresthesia is more likely to reflect a neurologic lesion such as a peripheral neuropathy or a compression neuropathy.

- Weakness and activity-induced muscle fatigue, particularly involving the eye and bulbar muscles, along with the limb musculature, should target the neuromuscular junction (i.e., myasthenia gravis). Exercise-induced muscle pain/cramping and weakness suggests a metabolic myopathy.

- Acute distal ascending weakness with loss of reflexes, often following an upper respiratory illness, may reflect Guillain-Barré syndrome, an acute inflammatory demyelinating polyneuropathy. A chronic demyelinating polyneuropathy can also occur.

- A mixed picture with muscle weakness, atrophy, and muscle fasciculation, combined with upper motor neuron signs, may reflect motor neuron disease, such as amyotrophic lateral sclerosis (ALS).

- Severe weakness, even quadriplegia, in a patient in the ICU may reflect a combination of critical illness myopathy/neuropathy, neuromuscular blockade, and drug toxicity.

PATIENT DEMOGRAPHICS

The peak age for inflammatory myositis is 45 to 55 years, but all ages can be affected, including children (DM). It is more common among women, with a female:male ratio of 2–3:1.

KEY QUESTIONS

1. What do you mean by "weakness"?

- Ask the patient to give an example of an activity limitation (e.g., getting off the toilet, getting off the floor, climbing stairs, holding up arms).

- Distinguish true weakness from fatigue, poor endurance, and weakness due to pain when attempting to perform an activity. Conditions that might cause functional weakness include: anemia; chronic heart, lung, or kidney disease; arthritis; and endocrinopathies.
- How fast has the weakness progressed? How have the symptoms changed since onset? Motor neuron disease is relentless and progressive over months to years with expanding areas of involvement; inflammatory myositis is insidious and progressive over weeks to months.
- Has there been a slow or intermittent decline in strength?
- The symptoms associated with neuromuscular junction disease fluctuate and tend to be worse later in the day.

2. What is the pattern and localization of weakness?

- What is the distribution of muscle involvement?
  - **Large muscles (getting up to walk):** Consider myositis/myopathy, myasthenia gravis.
  - **Small muscles (grasping and holding on to objects):** Consider polyneuropathy, compression neuropathy (if asymmetrical).
  - **Both large and small muscles:** Consider inclusion body myositis, motor neuron disease (progressive over time), demyelinating polyneuropathy.
- Are there any difficulties with vision (diplopia, ptosis), speech, or swallowing? Consider CNS or neuromuscular disease.
- Is there any pattern to the weakness such as worsening after exercise? Consider metabolic myopathy.

- Does the weakness worsen with repetitive action? Consider neuromuscular junction pathology.
- Is there any associated paresthesia, a bladder- or bowel-control problem, or incoordination? Consider central or peripheral nervous system disorders.

3. Is there pain associated with the weakness?
- If pain is intermittent and provoked by exercise, it may be due to metabolic myopathy; consider claudication in the setting of large vessel vasculitis.
- If it is sustained and more localized, it may be caused by nerve or muscle ischemia due to vasculitis.
- If it is acute, severe, highly localized, and associated with spinal pain, it may be due to radicular compression.
- If it is acute and generalized, consider rhabdomyolysis.
- Note that older patients with polymyalgia rheumatica have pain and stiffness, but do not have objective weakness (but certain resisted movements may be limited by pain).
- Myalgia may be present in some patients with inflammatory myositis.

4. Are there any constitutional symptoms such as fevers, night sweats, or weight loss?
- Consider systemic disease with associated inflammatory myositis.
- Consider malignancy (PM/DM may precede or follow the diagnosis of certain malignancies).

5. Are there any associated symptoms?
- Evolution of erythematous rash over the eyelids, extensor surfaces, and in sun-exposed areas

suggests DM. Shortness of breath may be due to interstitial lung disease in the context of DM or PM.

- Are there symptoms suggestive of connective tissue disease such as skin rash, joint pain, pleuritic chest pain, or Raynaud phenomenon? Consider systemic autoimmune disease with associated inflammatory myositis.

- Has there been recent weight gain associated with cold intolerance and dry skin or hair; or weight loss, excessive perspiration, and tremor? Are there features of hypercortisolism? Consider endocrine disease.

6. Has there been any recent severe illness?
Consider deconditioning, critical illness myopathy/ neuropathy, or rhabdomyolysis associated with severe viral illness, fever, and seizures.

7. Have any new medications been started in the last 6 months?
- Has the patient started statins, glucocorticoids, colchicine, etc.?

- Consider common drugs such as diuretics, which may cause hypokalemia and impairment of muscle function, as well over-the-counter medications and naturopathic medications.

8. Is past health remarkable for chronic disease?
- Ask about heart, lung, or kidney disease; chronic infection; anemia; arthritis; and malignancy. These might contribute to asthenia or functional weakness.

9. Is there any relevant family history?
- A family history of autoimmune or endocrine problems may provide a clue to the patient's problem.

- A history of neuromuscular disorders, or symptoms of exercise intolerance in family members, may indicate an inherited disorder.

10. What is the social history?

- Inquire about recreational drug exposure (especially cocaine) and sexual history (for hepatitis, HIV), and do a psychosocial review for stressors and depression.

- Is there a history of strenuous exercise and dehydration? Consider rhabdomyolysis.

Physical Examination

General appearance:

- Does the patient look well or unwell (i.e., short of breath, cyanotic, pale)?

- Is the patient able or not able to rise from a chair (without using upper extremities) and walk across the room?

- Does the patient show Gowers sign? (Patient attempts to rise from squatting or sitting on the floor by climbing up legs with hands—typically seen in children.)

Vital signs: These should be normal in most inflammatory myositis patients; vital signs outside normal range may reflect underlying disease or significant pulmonary involvement.

Skin and nails:

Findings in DM:

Heliotrope: a violaceous rash on the upper eyelids accompanied by swelling of the eyelid

Erythema in the shawl or V region of upper chest and back

Gottron papules: symmetrical scaly violaceous or erythematous rash over the extensor surface of MCP and PIP areas of the fingers

Periungual erythema due to nail-fold capillary abnormalities (vessel dropout or dilated loops)

"Mechanic's hands": painful rough hands with cracked skin on the tips and sides of the fingers

Calcinosis: subcutaneous calcification

Findings in amyopathic DM: These patients have skin changes only, with no muscle weakness (but they may develop severe lung involvement).

Findings in other conditions:

Systemic lupus erythematosus (SLE): butterfly rash

Scleroderma: tethered, thickened skin and telangiectasia

Vasculitis: purpura, leg ulcers, nodules

Dermatomyositis: Gottron sign (nonscaling erythema over MCP/PIP and other extensor areas)

Head and neck:

- Look for thyroid enlargement, lymphadenopathy, features of connective tissue disease (oral ulcers, dry mouth, parotid enlargement, etc.).
- Note any deviation of the tongue or fasciculations.

Pulmonary exam: Examine for tachypnea, crackles (interstitial lung disease of myositis), decreased expansion (restrictive lung disease), rubs, dullness (pleural disease).

Cardiovascular exam: Examine for elevated jugular venous pressure, gallop rhythm, edema (evidence of heart failure secondary to myositis), murmurs, symmetry of pulses, bruits.

Abdominal exam: Examine for masses (think malignancy), organomegaly, bruits.

Neurologic exam:

- Look for cranial nerve findings—e.g., ptosis (myasthenia gravis), bulbar weakness, tongue fasciculations (motor neuron disease).
- Facial weakness is seen with many muscular dystrophies.
- Oculomotor and facial weakness is not seen in inflammatory myositis.
- Test and grade muscle power:
  - **If weakness is asymmetrical:** Consider compression neuropathy, mononeuropathy/ mononeuritis multiplex, cerebrovascular disease, spinal cord disease, demyelinating disorders.
  - **If weakness is symmetrical:** If proximal, consider primary muscle diseases, including dystrophies (especially if isolated shoulder girdle), myasthenia gravis; if distal, consider peripheral neuropathy, motor neuron disease, myasthenia gravis, inclusion body myositis.

Weakness

MEDICAL RESEARCH COUNCIL GRADING FOR MUSCLE WEAKNESS

Grade 5	Normal strength
Grade 4	Muscle contraction possible against gravity and some resistance
Grade 3	Muscle contraction possible against gravity only
Grade 2	Muscle contraction possible only with gravity removed
Grade 1	Flicker of muscle contraction but no movement of extremity
Grade 0	No contraction

There is a wide range of muscle strength and +/− values are often added.

- If considering inflammatory myositis, specifically assess:
  - neck flexors (lifting head from bed when supine)
  - deltoids (shoulder abduction), triceps (elbow extension)
  - ability to rise from a squat or chair
  - iliopsoas (hip flexion)
  - quadriceps (knee extension)
  - truncal power (partial sit-up—i.e., raising the shoulders off the table, double leg lift from supine position)
- Muscle wasting may be seen in long-standing inflammatory myositis, muscular dystrophy.
- Assess grip strength, heel-and-toe walk (for inclusion body myositis, polyneuropathy, motor neuron disease).
- Assess reflexes:
  - Are they normal (e.g., myositis), increased (motor neuron disease, thyrotoxicosis), absent (e.g., polyneuropathy, inclusion body myositis), or delayed relaxation (e.g., hypothyroidism)?
  - Clonus may indicate motor neuron disease, upper spinal cord lesion.
- Look for sensory changes: dermatomal, peripheral nerve, spinal cord (look for a sensory level and include perineal sensation), or central.
- Look for gait abnormalities:
  - **Ataxic gait:** due to posterior column problems
  - **Foot drop:** due to L5 or peroneal nerve lesion, mono- or polyneuropathy, motor neuron disease

Musculoskeletal exam:
- Perform a screening joint examination: inflammatory joint findings may indicate SLE, mixed connective tissue disease, antisynthetase syndrome as part of PM/DM.

- True muscle weakness may be difficult to identify in the presence of arthritis.

Key Laboratory Investigations

INITIAL INVESTIGATIONS

CBC: Look for anemia (chronic disease, malignancy).

Creatinine, electrolytes, urinalysis: Consider looking for myoglobinuria. Expect these tests to produce findings with any muscle damage. These tests may also be helpful with metabolic myopathy in the setting of rhabdomyolysis.

CK: This is the most sensitive and specific test for muscle disease. The value may rise several weeks before muscle strength changes and will begin to fall before clinical improvement in strength after therapy for myositis is initiated. CK can be useful in monitoring response to therapy.

Other muscle enzymes, if available: Include aldolase, lactate dehydrogenase.

Extended chemistry: Include calcium, magnesium, phosphorus.

AST, ALT: Although less sensitive to muscle injury than CK, elevation of AST/ALT may indicate myositis rather than liver pathology.

Thyroid-stimulating hormone (TSH)

ESR, CRP: These may indicate an inflammatory process, but are neither sensitive nor specific.

ADDITIONAL TESTS FOR INFLAMMATORY MYOSITIS

Troponins, ECG, and/or 2D echocardiogram: Use these if there is a concern about myocardial involvement.

Chest X-ray: This assesses for interstitial lung disease, malignancy.

Autoantibodies:

- These include antinuclear antibody (ANA), extractable nuclear antigen, anti-double-stranded DNA (anti-dsDNA), complements.
- ANAs are found in up to 80% of patients with PM/DM.
- Several antibodies may reflect disease overlaps: anti-RNP (antiribonucleoprotein) with mixed connective tissue disease (SLE, PM, scleroderma); anti-Ku and anti-PM-Scl with scleroderma-PM overlaps.

Myositis-specific antibodies (present in up to one-third of patients):

- Anti-Jo-1 (anti-histadyl-tRNA synthetase) is present in 20% to 25% of PM/DM patients. It is associated with antisynthetase syndrome (PM/DM plus interstitial lung disease plus arthritis, Raynaud phenomenon, fever, and "mechanic's hands").
- Other antibodies associated with this syndrome include anti-PL7, anti-PL12, anti-EJ, and anti-OJ.

Other myositis-specific antibodies (difficult to obtain in standard laboratories):

- Anti-Mi-2 (anti-helicase) is present in acute onset of classic DM and associated with good response to treatment.
- Anti-SRP (anti-signal recognition peptide) is present in severe drug-resistant PM with cardiac involvement and necrotizing myopathy.
- Anti-P155/140 is present in juvenile DM and cancer in adult DM.
- Anti-HMGCR (anti-200/100) is present in 60% of necrotizing myopathy.
- Anti-MDA5 (anti-CADM-140) is present in DM with skin disease but no muscle weakness, and

acute progressive life-threatening interstitial lung disease. Consider especially in patients of Asian descent, or in patients with prominent respiratory symptoms.

Electromyography (EMG) and MRI:

- EMG and MRI are useful to objectively document the presence of a myopathy (and can be followed over time), as well as to ascertain the presence and severity of a neuropathy.
- Typical findings in inflammatory myopathy include small polyphasic action potentials; fibrillations, positive sharp waves, insertional irritability; repetitive high frequency action potentials.
- MRI can also be used to look for evidence of myositis (versus fatty tissue) and/or to localize a site for biopsy.

Muscle biopsy:

- This is the gold standard for diagnosis of myositis and should be considered in most patients. Biopsy a clinically weak muscle, but avoid any EMG site (where needle was inserted).
- Specimens must be appropriately handled for later testing (routine and electron microscopy, special biochemical tests, and testing for metabolic/inherited defects).
- Typical features of inflammatory myositis on biopsy include necrosis and regeneration of muscle fibres; variation of fibre size; endomysial inflammatory cell infiltration and perivascular inflammation with CD8+ T cells in PM; chronic inflammatory cell infiltrate in the perivascular and perifascicular areas with CD4+ T cells and B cells in DM.

Malignancy screening:
- This should be performed in patients presenting with PM/DM because of the temporal association between the conditions.
- A rational workup includes basic blood work and age- and gender-appropriate screening (e.g., colonoscopy in older individuals; mammogram, pelvic ultrasound in women; abdominal or pelvic ultrasound in most patients).

Skin biopsy: For DM, this may be redundant after workup of myositis, but in some circumstances may be sufficient for diagnosis.

Lactate, myoglobinuria screening: If you are considering metabolic myopathy, measuring lactate levels or screening for myoglobinuria may be helpful. EMG and forearm exercise test may also be useful in this workup.

ADDITIONAL TESTS FOR OTHER RHEUMATIC DISEASES AND VASCULITIS

Autoantibodies: Consider these tests, based on clinical evaluation.

Cryoglobulins, antineutrophil cytoplasmic antibodies

Nerve conduction studies: Vasculitic neuropathy may be identified by localizing anatomic lesions to the peripheral nerves (e.g., radial nerve in a patient presenting with wrist drop, peroneal nerve with foot drop).

ADDITIONAL TESTS FOR INFECTIOUS CAUSES

Hepatitis, HIV, HTLV1: Test for these as warranted.

ADDITIONAL TESTS FOR ENDOCRINOPATHIES

TSH, T3, T4, urinary cortisol, low-dose dexamethasone suppression, etc.: Consider these, as appropriate.

ADDITIONAL TESTS FOR PRIMARY NEUROLOGIC CONDITIONS

Brain CT scan or MRI, lumbar puncture: These may be required.

Nerve conduction studies: These ascertain whether there is axonal change ("conduction block" secondary to ischemia in the setting of vasculitis) or demyelinating disease (slowing of conduction and latencies—e.g., Guillain-Barré syndrome). It is possible to identify neuromuscular block seen in myasthenia gravis.

Differential Diagnosis

INFLAMMATORY MYOSITIS

Polymyositis (PM)
- Look for symmetric proximal muscle weakness.
- PM has constitutional symptoms (i.e., fever, weight loss, etc.).
- Patients may have: arthralgia or arthritis; dysphagia or gastroesophageal reflux disease; dyspnea.
- CK levels are typically greater than 1000 but less than 10 000.
- Look for myopathic change on EMG and characteristic muscle biopsy.

Dermatomyositis (DM)
This is similar to PM, but with typical rash or skin involvement.

PM/DM associated with malignancy
- This may present with a PM picture or as part of a paraneoplastic syndrome.
- Relative risk of cancer is increased 2 to 3 times in the presence of DM and less so in PM/DM.
- Most cancers are diagnosed within 2 years of

myositis and reflect those typical of the age group, with a slight increase in ovarian cancer.

PM/DM associated with connective tissue disease

Childhood DM

Inclusion body myositis

- This condition has more insidious onset with slower progression.
- It features proximal and distal weakness, muscle atrophy, and sometimes loss of reflexes.
- CK levels are lower than in PM/DM.
- Inclusion body myositis is more common in men.
- It can be confused with PM. A biopsy specimen is required to detect the hallmark finding of filamentous inclusions and vacuoles on electron microscopy.
- It has poor response to therapy.

Infection-related myositis

- HIV can be associated with general debility and a specific inflammatory myopathy.
- Trichinosis causes direct infection of muscle.
- Viral myositis is often acute and dramatic.

Other inflammatory myopathies

- Necrotizing autoimmune myopathy has very high CK. On biopsy, it presents with necrosis but no inflammation.
- Sarcoidosis can be associated with several types of myopathy, including a picture similar to PM, as well as a nodular form of inflammation.

TOXIC MYOPATHIES

Cocaine use has been associated with acute rhabdomyolysis.

DRUG-RELATED MYOPATHIES

- Colchicine can cause a myopathy, especially when used in the setting of renal failure.
- Statins are the most common cause of drug-related myopathy.
- Steroid-induced myopathy is common and this may lead to confusion when used in the treatment of myositis.

ENDOCRINE-RELATED MYOPATHIES

Both hypothyroidism and thyrotoxicosis can cause a proximal myopathy with elevated levels of CK.

INHERITED METABOLIC MYOPATHIES

- These conditions include disorders in lipid and glycogen metabolism, or abnormalities of mitochondrial electron transport chains.
- They often feature postexertion myalgia and weakness.

MUSCULAR DYSTROPHY (MD)

- Specific forms of MD can present in adults.
- Weakness tends to be proximal.
- Facial weakness may be present.
- MD can be confused with PM.
- It may present with elevated CK levels and little weakness. It may show mild inflammation on biopsy.
- MD does not respond to glucocorticoids.

NEUROLOGIC CAUSES

Possible neurologic causes include:

- upper motor neuron impairment (central, spinal cord)
- anterior horn cell disease

- peripheral nervous system lesions
- neuromuscular junction impairment

Initial Therapy for Inflammatory Myositis (PM/DM)

- Glucocorticoids should be started at a high dose, 1–1.5 mg/kg in divided doses. Administer IV therapy if there is significant dysphagia. Dose reduction can begin after 4 to 8 weeks, depending on the rate of improvement.
- CK normalizes before strength improves. Clinical improvement can be slow.
- Additional immunosuppressive agents may be needed, such as methotrexate or azathioprine.
- Other agents, including rituximab and IV immunoglobulin, may be required for more severe or resistant disease.
- Hydroxychloroquine should be added for cutaneous disease.
- Prophylaxis of glucocorticoid-induced osteoporosis is needed.
- Monitor for immunosuppressive toxicity (e.g., CBC, liver enzymes for azathioprine, methotrexate).
- Deterioration after initial response to treatment could be due to steroid myopathy. CK does not rise and EMG changes are different than in inflammatory disease. More rapid withdrawal of steroid and close monitoring may be indicated.
- Ensure workup is done to look for associated malignancy.
- Monitor the response of organs that may be secondarily involved in the setting of an associated connective tissue disease.

- Inclusion body myositis responds poorly to treatment, but a trial is warranted in most patients.

ACKNOWLEDGEMENT

Thanks to Dr. Sharon LeClercq, University of Calgary, who developed this chapter for the first edition of the *Canadian Residents' Rheumatology Handbook*, 2005.

Further Reading

Aggarwal R, Oddis CV. Therapeutic advances in myositis. *Curr Opin Rheumatol.* 2012;24(6):635–41. http://dx.doi.org/10.1097/BOR.0b013e328358ac72. Medline:22955021

Burr ML, Roos JC, Ostör AJK. Metabolic myopathies: a guide and update for clinicians. *Curr Opin Rheumatol.* 2008;20(6):639–47. http://dx.doi.org/10.1097/BOR.0b013e328315a05b. Medline:18946322

Smith EC, El-Gharbawy A, Koeberl DD. Metabolic myopathies: clinical features and diagnostic approach. *Rheum Dis Clin North Am.* 2011;37(2):201–17, vi. http://dx.doi.org/10.1016/j.rdc.2011.01.004. Medline:21444020

Younger DS. The myopathies. *Med Clin North Am.* 2003;87(4):899–907, ix. http://dx.doi.org/10.1016/S0025-7125(03)00030-0. Medline:12834153

Zong M, Lundberg IE. Pathogenesis, classification and treatment of inflammatory myopathies. *Nat Rev Rheumatol.* 2011;7(5):297–306. http://dx.doi.org/10.1038/nrrheum.2011.39. Medline:21468145

Weakness

4

Raynaud Phenomenon

DR. JANET POPE
UNIVERSITY OF WESTERN ONTARIO

KEY CONCEPTS

1. Raynaud phenomenon (RP) is reversible vasospasm of the digits with pallor and then cyanosis and/or rubor. Pallor must be present.

2. It is common: it affects at least 2% of the population, with onset usually in teens if idiopathic.

3. There are 2 types of RP:

   - **Primary:** Primary RP is idiopathic (not related to other diseases) and is not associated with structural vascular change or ischemic tissue damage.

   - **Secondary:** Secondary RP is related to other connective tissue diseases (CTDs) such as systemic lupus erythematosus (SLE), Sjögren syndrome, scleroderma (systemic sclerosis), rheumatoid arthritis (RA), polymyositis, undifferentiated CTD, mixed CTD. Patients who are antinuclear antibody (ANA) positive and anti-centromere antibody positive, and/or have nail fold (periungual) and superficial dilated capillaries, are more likely to develop a CTD at 5 years, such as limited cutaneous systemic sclerosis (limited subset of scleroderma).

4. Most primary RP will never need pharmacologic treatment. Keeping warm (hands, feet, and head) and smoking cessation are usually recommended.

5. Calcium channel blockers (CCBs) of the dihydropyridine type (e.g., nifedipine) are the main pharmacologic treatment for RP when warranted by symptoms.
6. The goal of pharmacologic treatment is to decrease the frequency, the severity, and the duration of attacks and to reduce or treat complications in those with secondary RP.
7. In secondary RP, there may be complications such as severe ischemia, ulcers, and loss of tissue.

History

PATIENT DEMOGRAPHICS

Primary RP

- Onset during teens is more common. People younger than 40 are most often affected.
- It occurs in 1% to 3% of the population.
- It has female preponderance.
- Patients may have a family history of RP and may also have migraines.

Secondary RP

- Secondary RP is associated with a disease (e.g., a CTD).
- Onset can occur at any age. Secondary RP especially accounts for older-onset RP.
- Secondary RP is often more severe than primary RP, and can be accompanied by digital ulcers and autoamputations.
- It occurs in most patients with scleroderma and in 10% to 20% of patients with Sjögren syndrome, SLE, and RA.
- It has female preponderance (because CTDs are more common in women).

- Patients may have a family history of RP and may also have migraines.

KEY QUESTIONS

These questions seek to establish whether the patient:

- is really experiencing RP
- has had complications, such as threatened digital ischemia or ulcers
- has an associated evolving CTD
- has a structural cause for RP

1. At what age did the RP begin?

Younger onset is more typical of primary RP.

2. Describe the attacks. Which digits are involved? How frequent and severe are the attacks?

- Episodic, well-demarcated pallor followed by cyanosis and rubor with rewarming is the classic RP episode. Cyanosis alone is not RP (see Figure 4.1).
- There may be associated pain. Increasing frequency and severity of attacks may indicate a secondary cause.

3. Have there been any ulcers, gangrene, or tissue loss?

Secondary sequelae suggest an underlying disease (secondary RP).

4. Are the symptoms unilateral?

RP that is very severe or only on 1 hand should alert you to a structural problem such as a unilateral stenosis, thrombosis or embolism, or vasculitis.

5. Are there any symptoms of CTD or other secondary causes?

- Ask about the following: oral ulcers, rash, photosensitivity, alopecia, dry eyes or mouth, gland

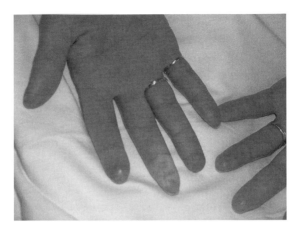

FIGURE 4.1. Raynaud phenomenon. Note blanching of (right third finger). This patient also has cyanosis (second and fourth digit) and multiple teangiectasia.

swelling, puffy fingers, tight skin, inflammation of joints, dysphagia, gastroesophageal reflux, kidney problems (glomerulonephritis, nephritic syndrome), serositis (pleurisy, pericarditis), subcutaneous lumps, numbness, tingling, shocking pain down an arm or leg (i.e., mononeuritis multiplex secondary to vasculitis), proximal weakness, severe headaches and/or ischemic arm pain (i.e., giant cell arteritis in older patients, Takayasu arteritis in younger patients).

- Has the patient had SLE, RA, or other CTD diagnosed previously?
- Are there any known hematologic disorders (e.g., paraproteins, cryoglobulins), malignancy, hypothyroidism, or atherosclerosis?
- Is there a smoking history?

6. Are any medications being taken?

Is the patient taking any therapy that might be contributing to RP? For example, patients receiving bleomycin as part of cancer chemotherapy can develop drug-induced RP.

7. What is the social history?

- Does the patient's occupation involve the use of vibration tools?
- Does the patient work in a cold environment?
- What is the smoking history (current or ever)?

8. Is there a family history of RP or CTD?

There is familial clustering of primary RP.

9. What is the functional status?

Does the RP interfere with the patient's life? Does the patient want or need medications to treat it?

Physical Examination

Vital signs: These are expected to be normal. Consider recording BP in each arm and checking pulses bilaterally to identify a possible structural problem.

Skin and nails:

- Look for rashes, evidence of photosensitivity, and puffy or tight skin (especially sclerodactyly): any of these findings may indicate an underlying CTD, especially scleroderma.

- Look for evidence of current or previous ischemia (e.g., digital pits): any of these findings may indicate an underlying CTD, especially scleroderma.

- Look for superficial dilated capillaries in the nail fold (dropout of capillaries with dilatation and hypertrophy of remaining vessels):
  - You can use an ophthalmoscope or otoscope to see red capillaries (lines) and/or hemorrhages at the periungual area.

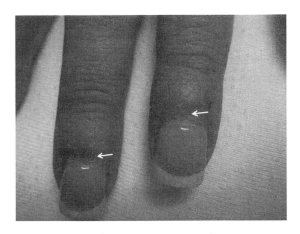

FIGURE 4.2. Nail-fold capillary changes in scleroderma (arrowheads).

- This is highly suggestive of secondary RP; see Figure 4.2.

Head and neck: Look for dry eyes and mouth, lymphadenopathy, salivary and/or lacrimal gland swelling, oral and nasal ulcers, and alopecia (i.e., changes associated with CTD).

Chest: Examine for effusions or rubs of serositis (uncommon) and bilateral basilar crackles of interstitial lung disease.

Abdomen: Findings are usually normal.

Neurologic exam: Findings are usually normal. Note, however:

- Some CTDs present with a stocking-and-glove peripheral neuropathy.
- Vasculitis may have an associated mononeuritis multiplex.

Musculoskeletal exam: Look for swollen joints and diffusely swollen fingers (puffy fingers of early scleroderma or mixed CTD).

Key Laboratory Investigations

- No tests are confirmatory.

- If you suspect secondary RP, check complete blood count, creatinine, and urinalysis to look for evidence of other target organ involvement as part of an underlying disease. Check ANA: patients who are ANA positive and have superficial dilated capillaries are more likely to develop a CTD (20% of these patients develop a CTD at 5 years, especially limited systemic scleroderma, and especially if ANA is anti-centromere antibody positive).

- Only if history or physical examination suggests a secondary cause would you do further testing, such as autoimmune serology, serum complements, antiphospholipid antibodies, cryoglobulins, chest X-ray, swallowing study, imaging of great vessels, and arterial Doppler.

Imaging

No studies are routinely useful in this setting (see "Key Laboratory Investigations").

Differential Diagnosis

Approach the differential diagnosis with the following distinctions in mind:

- whether the patient has RP or something else
- if it is RP, whether it is primary or secondary

DIFFERENTIAL DIAGNOSIS, IF NOT RP

Acrocyanosis

- This is characterized by persistent rather than episodic peripheral cyanosis with no associated tissue change.

- It is often associated with cold and clammy extremities and some swelling.
- It is typically idiopathic.
- It has secondary causes that overlap with causes of RP.

Exaggerated vasospasm

This presents as mottled or cold digits in normal young women.

Cryoglobulinemia or cold agglutinins

This presents as blue digits with no pallor. Consider cryoglobulinemia especially if lower extremities are involved.

Perniosis (chilblains)*

- This presents as erythematous or blue small plaques or nodules on the toes or fingers, especially at the tips. Patients often report pain and cold digits and may have distal cyanosis.
- The condition is similar to frostbite or trench foot, where cold and dampness damage cutaneous capillaries.
- It may be associated erythema, blisters, and pruritus.
- Half of cases are idiopathic and half are associated with a CTD such as SLE.

Thromboangiitis obliterans (Buerger disease)*

Suspect this conditions if the patient has severely ischemic digit(s), with no vasospastic component and a smoking history.

Complex regional pain syndrome

The patient's extremity may be cool and mottled, but not consistent with classic RP.

Note: These conditions may be associated with true RP.

Raynaud

DIFFERENTIAL DIAGNOSIS FOR A SECONDARY CAUSE, IF RP

Drug-induced RP

Drugs that can cause RP include:

- ergotamine and other migraine medications
- chemotherapy (e.g., bleomycin)
- over-the-counter decongestants
- exogenous estrogen therapies (some)
- cocaine, amphetamines

Structural RP

- **In large and medium vessels,** consider:
  - thoracic outlet syndrome
  - brachiocephalic trunk disease (e.g., Takayasu vasculitis or giant cell arteritis)

- **In small arteries and arterioles,** consider:
  - CTD
  - other autoimmune disease (e.g., RA)
  - cold injury (frostbite)
  - vibration injury (e.g., jackhammer operators)

Hematologic RP

Consider:

- cryoglobulinemia and other paraproteins (hyperviscosity)
- cold agglutinins
- polycythemia rubra vera
- antiphospholipid antibody syndrome

Initial Therapy

NONPHARMACOLOGIC (UNPROVEN)

- Stay warm (avoid cold, use warm clothing, use mittens rather than gloves, wear a hat, and use hand and foot warmers).
- Stop smoking and avoid stress.

PHARMACOLOGIC

Dihydropyridine calcium channel blockers (CCBs)

- These are the mainstay of therapy if prescription medication is necessary, and are often used as needed in winter or with season change.
- Dihydropyridine CCBs include nifedipine (long acting or short acting), amlodipine, felodipine, and nicardipine.
- Long-acting preparations have less potential for hypotension as a side effect.
- Dose can be increased if drug is tolerated and efficacy is not sufficient after a few days to 1 to 2 weeks of therapy.
- **Topical nitrates:** A low dose applied sparingly to the digital web spaces can be effective. (Oral treatments are more apt to give side effects, including headache and hypotension.)

OTHER OPTIONS

If CCBs fail or are not tolerated

Consider:

- angiotensin II blockers such as losartan
- selective serotonin reuptake inhibitors (SSRIs) such as fluoxetine
- other CCBs (possibly diltiazem, but not verapamil)
  - These usually do not provide sufficient benefit.
  - They are used only if dihydropyridine CCBs are not tolerated or if there is another reason, such as cardiac disease, to warrant diltiazem use.

If severe or complicated RP

Consider:

- phosphodiesterase 5 (PDE5) inhibitors (such as sildenafil, tadalafil, vardenafil)

Raynaud

- IV prostacyclin (prostaglandin I2) (iloprost) or epoprostenol for severe digital ischemia or complications
- combination treatment (sometimes used—e.g., CCB with PDE5 inhibitor)
  - Note that combination treatment creates a higher risk of adverse events such as symptomatic hypotension.

Possible option
Although not routinely used to treat RP, beta blockers with CCBs may help.

- It may be appropriate to prescribe a CCB for a patient who already takes a beta blocker.
- Note that beta blockers alone do not treat RP.

Rarely used option
Because of hypotension, some effective drugs are not used:

- alpha blockers (e.g., prazosin)
- adrenergic neuron blocker (guanethidine)
- pentoxifylline (negative data)

Surgery or injections
These include:

- stellate or lumbar ganglion sympathetic blocks
- selective local sympathectomies
- implantable devices to decrease sympathetic nerve stimulation

Unknown benefit
Some possible but unproven therapies include:

- botulinum toxin A (Botox) injections near digital arteries
- ketanserin (positive and negative data)
- biofeedback (some negative and positive trial data)

- low-level laser
- *Ginkgo biloba* in primary RP (some positive data, but inferior to nifedipine)
- probucol (antioxidant)
- fish oil

ADJUNCTIVE THERAPY

- For digital ischemia, consider use of ASA (it is unknown if other antiplatelet therapies are effective).
- For thrombus (such as in antiphospholipid antibody syndrome), consider use of low-molecular-weight heparin, warfarin, or other oral anticoagulant drugs.
- Consider analgesics for ischemic pain (morphine is preferred due to vasodilation).
- Rest the digit (decrease demand).

TREATMENT SPECIFIC TO SCLERODERMA

In secondary RP associated with systemic sclerosis, data support some treatments of digital ulcers and other treatments for prevention of subsequent ulcers.

Healing of digital ulcers
Therapies include:

- CCBs (nifedipine)
- IV iloprost
- PDE5 inhibitors (e.g., sildenafil, tadalafil)

Prevention of digital ulcers
Therapies include:

- atorvastatin (high dose)
- bosentan
- therapies indicated for healing of digital ulcers (probably)

Raynaud

Adjunctive treatment of digital ulcers

- Consider ASA to improve blood flow.
- Treat pain.
- Treat digital infections if present with antibiotics.

Further Reading

Chung L, Shapiro L, Fiorentino D, et al. MQX-503, a novel formulation of nitroglycerin, improves the severity of Raynaud phenomenon: a randomized, controlled trial. *Arthritis Rheum.* 2009;60(3):870–7. http://dx.doi.org/10.1002/art.24351. Medline:19248104

Kowal-Bielecka O, Landewé R, Avouac J, et al; EUSTAR co-authors. EULAR recommendations for the treatment of systemic sclerosis: a report from the EULAR Scleroderma Trials and Research group (EUSTAR). *Ann Rheum Dis.* 2009;68(5):620–8. http://dx.doi.org/10.1136/ard.2008.096677. Medline:19147617

Malenfant D, Catton M, Pope JE. The efficacy of complementary and alternative medicine in the treatment of Raynaud phenomenon: a literature review and meta-analysis. *Rheumatology (Oxford).* 2009;48(7):791–5. http://dx.doi.org/10.1093/rheumatology/kep039. Medline:19433434

Malenfant D, Summers K, Seney S, et al. Results of a pilot randomized placebo-controlled trial in Raynaud phenomenon with St. John's wort: detecting changes in angiogenic cytokines when RP improves. ISRN Rheumatol [Internet]. 2011 [cited 2011 Jun 27]; 2011: Article ID 580704 [6 p.]. Epub 2011 Sep 12. Available from: http://www.hindawi.com/journals/isrn/2011/580704/cta/.

Pope J. Raynaud phenomenon (primary). *Clin Evid (Online).* 2013;2013:1119. Medline:24112969

Pope J, Fenlon D, Thompson A, et al. Iloprost and cisaprost for Raynaud phenomenon in progressive systemic sclerosis. 1998 Apr 27. In: The Cochrane Database of Systematic Reviews [Internet]. Hoboken (NJ): John Wiley & Sons, Ltd. c2009 Available from: http://onlinelibrary.wiley.com/doi/10.1002/14651858.CD000953/abstract Article No.: CD000953.

Pope JE. The diagnosis and treatment of Raynaud phenomenon: a practical approach. *Drugs.* 2007;67(4):517–25. http://dx.doi.org/10.2165/00003495-200767040-00003. Medline:17352512

Pope JE, Al-Bishri J, Al-Azem H, et al. The temporal relationship of Raynaud phenomenon and features of connective tissue disease in rheumatoid arthritis. *J Rheumatol.* 2008;35(12):2329–33. http://dx.doi.org/10.3899/jrheum.071025. Medline:18843783

Thompson AE, Pope JE. Calcium channel blockers for primary Raynaud phenomenon: a meta-analysis. *Rheumatology (Oxford).* 2005;44(2):145–50. http://dx.doi.org/10.1093/rheumatology/keh390. Medline:15546967

Thompson AE, Shea B, Welch V, et al. Calcium-channel blockers for Raynaud phenomenon in systemic sclerosis. *Arthritis Rheum.* 2001;44(8):1841–7. http://dx.doi.org/10.1002/1529-0131(200108)44:8<1841::AID-ART322>3.0.CO;2-8. Medline:11508437

Tingey T, Shu J, Smuczek J, Pope J. Meta-analysis of healing and prevention of digital ulcers in systemic sclerosis. *Arthritis Care Res (Hoboken)*. 2013; 65(9):1460–71. http://dx.doi.org/10.1002/acr.22018. Medline:23554239

Walker KM, Pope J; participating members of the Scleroderma Clinical Trials Consortium (SCTC); Canadian Scleroderma Research Group (CSRG). Treatment of systemic sclerosis complications: what to use when first-line treatment fails--a consensus of systemic sclerosis experts. *Semin Arthritis Rheum*. 2012;42(1):42–55. http://dx.doi.org/10.1016/j.semarthrit.2012.01.003. Medline:22464314

Raynaud

The Patient Who Is Systemically Unwell

Is It Vasculitis?

DR. PATRICK LIANG
UNIVERSITÉ DE SHERBROOKE

KEY CONCEPTS

1. You should suspect a systemic vasculitis in the following clinical scenarios:
   - multiple organ involvement that is difficult to explain by a single disease process
   - systemic symptoms (e.g., fever, weight loss, cachexia) that cannot be explained after usual investigations
   - organ ischemia or infarction (myocardial infarction, bowel infarction), or hemorrhage (e.g., ruptured aneurysm)
   - a common condition (e.g., myocardial infarction, congestive heart failure) in an uncommon age group

2. The presentation of systemic vasculitides varies according to the **size and distribution of the blood vessels** in the disease process. A useful classification based on the size of vessels that are predominantly involved is shown in Figure 5a.1. Implicit in this classification is that features of vasculitis of a given vessel size may overlap with those from a different vessel size category. For example, a medium-size

vasculitis may demonstrate findings of small-vessel involvement as well, although these would not be the dominant findings. Table 5a.1 provides a summary of clinical features based on vessel size.

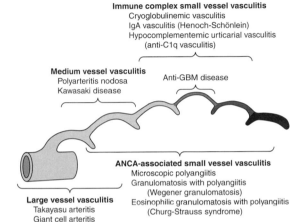

Immune complex small vessel vasculitis
Cryoglobulinemic vasculitis
IgA vasculitis (Henoch-Schönlein)
Hypocomplementemic urticarial vasculitis
(anti-C1q vasculitis)

Medium vessel vasculitis
Polyarteritis nodosa
Kawasaki disease

Anti-GBM disease

ANCA-associated small vessel vasculitis
Microscopic polyangiitis
Granulomatosis with polyangiitis
(Wegener granulomatosis)
Eosinophilic granulomatosis with polyangiitis
(Churg-Strauss syndrome)

Large vessel vasculitis
Takayasu arteritis
Giant cell arteritis

FIGURE 5a.1. Classification of vasculitis based on vessel size. Abbreviations: ANCA, antineutrophil cytoplasmic antibody; GBM, glomerular basement membrane. Used with permission from Jennette et al.[1]

TABLE 5a.1. Key clinical features of vasculitis by size of vessel involved

Organ system	Large vessel vasculitis (aorta and main branches)	Medium vessel vasculitis (main visceral arteries and their proximal branches)	Small vessel vasculitis (small parenchymal arteries, arterioles, capillaries, postcapillary venules)
Skin	Rare	Livedo reticularis	Purpura (palpable or not)
		Skin ulceration	Small necrotic papules
		Erythema nodosum	Vesicles
			Superficial ulcerations
Peripheral vascular	Asymmetry of pulses, BP in limbs (patients may experience claudication)	Digit necrosis	Splinter hemorrhages
			DVT (increased risk with SVV)

(Continued)

Vasculitis

TABLE 5a.1. (Continued)

Organ system	Large vessel vasculitis (aorta and main branches)	Medium vessel vasculitis (main visceral arteries and their proximal branches)	Small vessel vasculitis (small parenchymal arteries, arterioles, capillaries, postcapillary venules)
Cardiac	Murmurs (AI due to dilatation of aortic root)	Coronary ischemia	Pericarditis, myocarditis/cardiomyopathy, especially EGPA
Visceral vasculature	Aneurysms Stenoses (e.g., renovascular hypertension, mesenteric ischemia)	Microaneurysms (may have secondary rupture and hemorrhage) Mesenteric ischemia Renal infarcts or AKI (ischemic) Hypertension	GI (uncommon) Glomerulonephritis
Pulmonary	Pulmonary artery involvement	Generally spared (except with BD and pulmonary artery involvement)	Alveolar hemorrhage (GPA and MPA) Asthma (EGPA) Upper airway involvement (GPA and EGPA)
Central nervous system	Strokes/TIA (thromboembolic)		Cranial nerve abnormalities Mass lesions in CNS
Peripheral nervous system		Mononeuritis multiplex	Mononeuritis multiplex

Abbreviations: AI, aortic insufficiency; AKI, acute kidney injury; DVT, deep vein thrombosis; SVV, small vessel vasculitis; TIA, transient ischemic attack.

According to the revised International Chapel Hill Consensus Conference nomenclature of vasculitides,[1] vessel size may be defined as follows:

- **Large:** aorta and/or its major branches (e.g., carotid, subclavian, axillary, brachial, celiac, femoral, and proximal renal arteries)
- **Medium**: main visceral arteries and their proximal branches (e.g., coronary arteries,

hepatic arteries, intraparenchymal renal arteries)

- **Small:** small intraparenchymal arteries, arterioles, capillaries, and venules

3. A complete history and physical examination are instrumental to the diagnosis. A high index of suspicion is required to diagnose systemic vasculitis.

4. Laboratory results, as well as electromyography (EMG) and diagnostic imaging modalities, are helpful in differentiating forms of vasculitis from each other and from other diagnostic possibilities.

5. Biopsy, when possible, is extremely important to confirm the diagnosis, help differentiate forms of systemic vasculitis, and support therapeutic decisions. Biopsy should be performed in an involved organ. Blind biopsies have a low diagnostic yield and thus should be avoided.

6. The outcome of systemic vasculitis can be catastrophic and investigations and diagnosis must be completed in an expedient fashion.

Vasculitis

ABBREVIATIONS USED IN THIS CHAPTER FOR VASCULITIS SYNDROMES

AAV: antineutrophil cytoplasmic antibody–associated vasculitides (ANCA-associated vasculitides)

BD: Behçet disease

EGPA: eosinophilic granulomatosis with polyangiitis (formerly Churg-Strauss syndrome)

GCA: giant cell arteritis

GPA: granulomatosis with polyangiitis (formerly Wegener granulomatosis)

HSP: Henoch-Schönlein purpura

HUVS: hypocomplementemic urticarial vasculitis syndrome

KD: Kawasaki disease

MPA: microscopic polyangiitis

PAN: polyarteritis nodosa
TA: Takayasu arteritis

History

- Symptoms obtained in the history may be nonspecific, but the **pattern or constellation of symptoms** in a patient may help to raise suspicion of a systemic vasculitis and may also help differentiate forms of systemic vasculitis (Table 5a.1).

- A history of drug exposure, hepatitis, or high-risk behaviours, or a previous diagnosis of a connective tissue disease (CTD), is important to ascertain.

- Complaints of fatigue, weakness, fever, arthralgias, abdominal pain, hypertension, renal insufficiency, and neurologic dysfunction are particularly common.

PATIENT DEMOGRAPHICS

Characteristic epidemiologic features of individual vasculitic syndromes are shown in Table 5a.2.

KEY QUESTIONS

1. Are there fevers?

- Fevers can be a feature of any systemic vasculitis or CTD, especially systemic lupus erythematosus (SLE), PAN, GPA, MPA, TA, GCA.

- It is most important to rule out more common causes of fever and mimickers of vasculitis, including:
  - infections (bacterial, viral, fungal, mycobacterial)
  - systemic causes (bacterial endocarditis, atrial myxoma, sarcoidosis)

2. Is there weight loss?

- Weight loss can be a feature of any systemic vasculitis, especially PAN, GPA, EGPA, MPA.

TABLE 5a.2. Characteristic features of individual vasculitic syndromes

Vasculitis	Sex	Age	Ethnic association	Clinical characteristics
KD	♀ = ♂	Most patients: > 3 months and < 5 years	Asian	Persistent fever, strawberry tongue, palmar desquamation, conjunctivitis, coronary artery aneurysm
HSP	♀ = ♂	Most patients < 18 years; uncommon in adults (incidence ≈ 1–2 /10⁶)	—	Most common systemic vasculitis in children; palpable purpura, abdominal pain, arthritis, IgA nephropathy
Cogan syndrome	♀ = ♂	Young adult	—	Keratitis, vestibulo-auditory loss, aortitis
TA	♀ > ♂	< 30 years	Asian/ Hispanic	Pulselessness, fever, carotidynia, limb claudication, abdominal pain, hypertension, bruits
BD	♀ = ♂	< 35 years	Middle Eastern	Recurrent oral/genital ulcers, superficial and deep thrombophlebitis, uveitis (anterior, posterior, panuveitis), folliculitis, subcutaneous nodules, arthritis (usually mono- or oligoarticular, knees, ankles, elbows, wrists), CNS involvement
PAN	♀ < ♂	Middle age	—	Weight loss, fever, myalgias (can be severe), neuropathy, abdominal pain/ infarction, hypertension, renal insufficiency from nonglomerulonephritis causes (renal artery or parenchymal vessel involvement), livedo racemosa, subcutaneous nodules, skin ulceration, chronic hepatitis B (rare), usually **no** lung involvement, negative ANCA

(incidence ≈ 1–2 /10⁶) noted as $\approx 1\text{–}2\,/10^6$

Vasculitis

(Continued)

TABLE 5a.2. (Continued)

Vasculitis	Sex	Age	Ethnic association	Clinical characteristics
GPA	♀ = ♂	Middle age	—	Chronic sinusitis, otitis media, purpura, pulmonary infiltrates and nodules, arthralgias and arthritis, GN, cANCA/anti-PR3
MPA	♀ = ♂	Middle age	—	Pulmonary hemorrhage, GN, purpura, peripheral neuropathy, pANCA/anti-MPO
EGPA	♀ = ♂	Middle age	—	Asthma (often late onset), sinusitis/polyps, eosinophilia, pulmonary infiltrates, peripheral neuropathy (mononeuritis multiplex), arthralgias and arthritis, pANCA/anti-MPO (up to 50% of patients)
Isolated cerebral angiitis	♀ = ♂	Middle age	—	Headache, symptoms reflective of focal and diffuse CNS abnormalities, absence of systemic involvement, abnormal CSF, abnormal cerebral imaging
Mixed cryo-globulinemia	♀ < ♂	Adult	—	GN, arthritis, purpura, peripheral neuropathy, hepatitis C, type II mixed cryoglobulins (high rheumatoid factor titre), low C3 and especially C4
GCA	♀ > ♂	> 50 years (most > 65)	Northern European	Polymyalgia rheumatica, new headaches, scalp tenderness, visual loss, diplopia, jaw claudication, upper extremity claudication, asymmetry of pulse/BP, elevated ESR and CRP

Abbreviations: ANCA, antineutrophil cytoplasmic antibody; cANCA, cytoplasmic ANCA; GN, glomerulonephritis; anti-MPO, antimyeloperoxidase; pANCA, perinuclear ANCA; anti-PR3, anti-proteinase 3.

- Consider more common causes and mimickers of vasculitis first:
  - primary metabolic and systemic disorders (thyroid disease, diabetes, malabsorption, neoplasia, chronic infection)
  - psychiatric conditions (anorexia, depression)

3. Does the patient have arthralgias or arthritis?

- This is very common in CTDs, as well as systemic vasculitides.
- Consider SLE, GPA, EGPA, PAN, HSP, MPA, and BD.
- The pattern of joint symptoms in systemic vasculitis is variable (small joint polyarthritis to larger joint mono- or oligoarthritis) and so the pattern of joint pain is unlikely to help differentiate among CTDs or systemic vasculitides. Some suggestive patterns are shown in Table 5a.3.
- Consider also common arthritides, such as rheumatoid arthritis (RA), psoriatic, spondylarthritis.
- Consider infectious causes (e.g., viral or bacterial infection) and other systemic diseases (e.g., sarcoidosis, inflammatory bowel disease).

4. Is there headache?

- Headache is a common nonspecific symptom in patients generally, unless it is associated with scalp tenderness or localized temporal or occipital pain and/or jaw claudication (think GCA).
- Consider GCA, SLE, BD, isolated cerebral angiitis, and AAV.
- Eye involvement (anterior and posterior scleritis), and involvement of ear, nose, and/or throat, may manifest as headache.

5. Is there Raynaud phenomenon?

- Most often Raynaud phenomenon (RP) is idiopathic. Look for evidence of secondary RP (see chapter 4).

Vasculitis

TABLE 5a.3. Patterns of joint involvement characteristic of certain forms of vasculitis

Vasculitis type	Expected pattern of joint pain
GCA	PMR occurs in up to 40% of patients.
	Peripheral arthritis is uncommon in GCA (negatively associated with GCA).
AAV	This presents as short-lived (days) intermittent or migratory mono- or oligoarthritis.
	It can look like RA.
Rheumatoid vasculitis	Patients have long-standing, seropositive, nodular, erosive RA that may be inactive at the time of vasculitis.
HSP	This involves large joints, frequently the knees and ankles, with painful edema.
	The joint pain syndrome resolves within 4 weeks.
BD	This typically involves large joints—knees, ankles, elbows, wrists—in a mono- or oligoarticular pattern.

Abbreviations: PMR, polymyalgia rheumatica; RA, rheumatoid arthritis.

- Consider association with CTDs (SLE, systemic sclerosis, Sjögren syndrome, dermatomyositis).
- Consider PAN and cryoglobulinemia.

6. Is there neuropathic pain, polyneuropathy, or mononeuritis multiplex?

- First consider other causes for neuropathy, including:
  - diabetes mellitus, alcohol, B_{12} deficiency
  - collagen vascular disease (e.g., Sjögren syndrome, SLE)
  - infection (e.g., Lyme disease; mycobacterial infection such as leprosy; viruses such as hepatitis B, C, HIV)
  - neoplasm (mostly hematological)
  - sarcoidosis
  - multiple compression injury

- **Mononeuritis multiplex should raise the possibility of vasculitis if there are no other apparent causes.**
- Consider PAN, GPA, EGPA, MPA, and cryoglobulinemic vasculitis. (Peripheral polyneuropathy is more common in cryoglobulinemic vasculitis than mononeuritis multiplex, as seen in other vasculitides.)

7. Is there limb claudication?

This may relate to arterial insufficiency in conditions such as TA, GCA, or arterial thrombosis of BD, or antiphospholipid antibody syndrome.

8. Is there cognitive or behavioural change?

- Consider systemic illness, sepsis, metabolic causes, SLE.
- Consider BD, isolated cerebral angiitis (primary angiitis of the CNS).

9. Is there vision loss or reduction, and/or red and painful eye?

- Consider primary ocular diseases (e.g., uveitis, peripheral ulcerative keratitis, retinitis, retinal detachment, sarcoidosis).
- Consider particularly GCA (older individuals), TA, BD, GPA, Cogan syndrome, and HUVS.

10. Does the patient have sinusitis or upper respiratory tract symptoms?

- Consider infectious and allergic causes first. Also consider **cocaine-induced lesions.**
- Consider GPA, EGPA, and Cogan syndrome.

11. Is there chest pain, cough, shortness of breath, or hemoptysis?

- Consider other systemic diseases or infections (e.g., pneumonia, bronchiectasis, pulmonary embolus, neoplasia).

Vasculitis

- Consider pulmonary-renal syndrome: SLE, GPA, MPA, Goodpasture syndrome (see chapter 15).
- Consider TA and BD (frank hemoptysis due to pulmonary artery vasculitis).
- Consider KD in children.
- Stridor could mean cricoarytenoid involvement (RA), subglottic stenosis (GPA), or laryngo-tracheomalacia (relapsing polychondritis).
- Recent-onset asthma (especially with eosinophilia) greatly increases concern for EGPA.

12. Is there abdominal pain?
- Consider more common causes first (peptic ulcer disease, diverticulitis, peritonitis, surgical abdomen) and other systemic conditions (e.g., inflammatory bowel disease).
- Bowel ischemia or infarction may be the cause of abdominal pain in a patient with other multisystem involvement that could suggest a systemic vasculitis. Also consider thromboembolic conditions and segmental arterial mediolysis (especially in setting of celiac disease, hepatic disorders, mesenteric distribution).
- Consider PAN, HSP, SLE, BD, and TA.

Physical Examination

The diagnosis of systemic vasculitis is often delayed because its clinical features are seen in several disorders. Some physical signs are particularly suggestive (e.g., mononeuritis multiplex, palpable purpura). The pattern of organ involvement may suggest a certain vasculitis (e.g., hemoptysis and renal disease— GPA, MPA, SLE, Goodpasture syndrome).

Always consider clues indicating infection or nonvasculitic systemic diseases.

General appearance: Does the patient look unwell or acutely ill?

Vital signs:
Look for:

- tachycardia (think bleeding, respiratory distress, etc.)
- tachypnea (think pulmonary involvement)
- hypertension (think glomerulonephritis: GPA, MPA, SLE; or nonglomerulonephritis: TA, PAN)

If TA or GCA is suspected, be sure to:

- Check the symmetry of pulses and BP in limbs.
- Listen for bruits.

Head and neck:
- In the mouth, look for:
  - oral ulcers (think BD, SLE)
  - "strawberry" tongue in children (KD)

- In the nose, sinus, and ear, look for:
  - sinusitis, nasal congestion, polyps (GPA, EGPA—always consider coexistent infection)
  - nasal crusting (GPA)
  - nasal septum perforation (GPA, cocaine-induced midline destructive lesion, midline granuloma)
  - vertigo or hypoacousia (GPA; Cogan syndrome, Susac syndrome; BD; relapsing polychondritis)

- In the eyes, look for:
  - optic neuropathy (GCA, SLE, Sjögren syndrome, others such as sarcoidosis)
  - uveitis (BD, AAV, others such as sarcoidosis)

- scleritis (GPA, SLE, relapsing polychondritis, others such as RA)

Chest:
Look for:

- hemoptysis (GPA, MPA, Goodpasture syndrome, SLE, cryoglobulinemic vasculitis, BD, TA)
- wheezing, asthma (EGPA)
- consolidation (GPA, MPA, EGPA, Goodpasture syndrome, sarcoidosis, SLE)
- stridor (GPA with upper airway involvement, relapsing polychondritis)

Note that PAN seldom, if ever, involves the lungs.

Abdomen:
- There may be findings if the condition has GI involvement.
- Check for bruits (TA).

Cardiac exam:
- Check for murmurs (bacterial endocarditis as mimicker of vasculitis).
- Assess for elevated jugular venous pressure, gallops, peripheral edema, and pericardial involvement.
- Evidence of cardiac involvement has serious prognostic implications in vasculitis.
- Note that peripheral edema may be a sign of hypoalbuminemia secondary to glomerulonephritis in small vessel vasculitis (AAV, HSP, cryoglobulinemic vasculitis, Goodpasture syndrome, SLE).

Skin:
- Palpable purpura suggests small vessel vasculitis, including:
  - AAV

- immune complex small vessel vasculitis (HUVS, mixed cryoglobulinemia, HSP, SLE and other CTD, infection-associated vasculitis)
- drug-related vasculitis

- The following findings suggest medium-sized muscular artery vasculitis: livedo reticularis; deep, punched-out ulcers; and subcutaneous nodules. Consider:
  - PAN
  - rheumatoid vasculitis
  - SLE or antiphospholipid antibody syndrome

- The following symptoms suggest BD: genital (and oral) ulcers, folliculitis, erythema nodosum-like lesions, superficial thrombophlebitis, pathergy (e.g., pustule formation at venipuncture sites).

- For findings of periungual erythema:
  - Consider systemic vasculitides (e.g., GPA, EGPA).
  - Consider CTDs (e.g., SLE; dermatomyositis or polymyositis; systemic sclerosis; mixed connective tissue disease). Note, however, that periungual erythema is nonspecific for CTDs.

Musculoskeletal exam: Although distribution and patterns vary and are thus less specific, some vasculitic syndromes are accompanied by suggestive musculoskeletal features (see Table 5a.3).

Central nervous system:

- Look for peripheral neuropathy/mononeuritis multiplex (SLE, PAN, AAV, cryoglobulinemic vasculitis, Sjögren syndrome).

- CNS involvement may manifest in diverse ways, but is usually not the initial or sole manifestation of systemic vasculitides.

Vasculitis

- Look for signs of **focal disease** (e.g., transient ischemic attack, stroke, partial seizures, movement disorders, optic neuropathy, myelopathy, cranial neuropathy) and **diffuse disease** (e.g., cognitive or behavioural disorders, encephalopathy, meningitis).

- Most vasculitis syndromes involve the CNS, either directly or indirectly, by way of secondary metabolic, infectious, drug-related, or thromboembolic complications.

- Consider primary angiitis of the CNS and systemic vasculitic syndromes, in particular BD, SLE, Sjögren syndrome, AAV, and GCA. Some characteristic presentations include:
  - meningeal involvement and cranial neuropathies (GPA)
  - acute ischemic optic neuropathy (GCA)
  - dominant brainstem involvement (e.g., cranial neuropathy, pyramidal signs, behavioural changes, neuro-otologic signs) (BD)
  - dural sinus thrombosis (BD)
  - pseudotumour cerebri (HUVS)—note glucocorticoid treatment as a possible risk factor

Key Laboratory Investigations
CBC:

- WBC count is frequently elevated with neutrophilia in systemic vasculitis (in contrast to leukopenia seen in active SLE or in immunosuppressive drug-related complications).

- Consider sepsis.

- Eosinophilia is seen in association with EGPA.

Creatinine and urinalysis: Look for proteinuria or active renal sediment suggesting a glomerulonephritis and reduction in glomerular filtration rate. **These tests should be done in every patient with a suspicion of vasculitis: renal involvement can progress rapidly.**

Investigations to assess for infection: Consider cultures of blood, urine, ulcers, bone marrow, and CSF. Provide biopsy material as appropriate.

ESR, CRP: Findings are nonspecific, but frequently elevated.

Antinuclear antibodies: This is useful as a screen for SLE, but there is an increased incidence of positive results in other systemic vasculitides. Antibodies against extractable nuclear antigens and anti-double-stranded DNA (anti-dsdsDNA) antibodies may help to identify SLE, other specific CTDs, or overlap syndromes.

Rheumatoid factor: This test is nonspecific, although it may be positive in rheumatoid vasculitis, cryoglobulinemic vasculitis, and infection-related vasculitis.

C3, C4:

- Levels are reduced in cryoglobulinemia and some patients with active SLE, HUVS, and rheumatoid vasculitis.
- Levels are occasionally reduced in HSP.
- Note that levels may also be reduced in infection-related glomerulonephritis.

Cryoglobulins:

- Cryoglobulins are immunoglobulins found in serum that precipitate at below 37°C. Blood must be drawn into a warmed tube and kept warm in transit to the laboratory, where it will be centrifuged at 37°C before removing the serum to a 4°C refrigerator for 1 week to look for cryoprecipitates.

- Immunoglobulins may be monoclonal (type 1), as seen in myeloma and Waldenstrom macroglobulinemia; a mixture of monoclonal and polyclonal immunoglobulin (type 2); or polyclonal (type 3). Types 2 and 3 may be seen in CTD and in viral infections such as hepatitis C and HIV.

Hepatitis serology: Of patients with mixed cryoglobulinemia, approximately 90% have positive hepatitis C serological results. There is an increased association of hepatitis B infection and PAN, though the association is rarer now than it was in the past.

Antineutrophil cytoplasmic antibodies (ANCAs):

- ANCAs are assayed by indirect immunofluorescence (IIF) and confirmed by enzyme-linked immunosorbent assay (ELISA) testing for vasculitis-associated antibody specificities. They are seen in many patients with a small-vessel systemic vasculitis (see also chapter 10).

- Two patterns of ANCA positivity are seen:
  - **Anti-proteinase 3 (Anti-PR3):** This antibody pattern, found by ELISA, correlates with cytoplasmic staining by immunofluorescence assay (IFA) (cANCA—i.e., cytoplasmic ANCA). It is the most specific antibody pattern for GPA (80% to 95% of patients). It is occasionally seen in patients who have clinical diagnoses of MPA, EGPA, and Goodpasture syndrome.

- **Antimyeloperoxidase (anti-MPO):** This antibody pattern, found by ELISA, correlates with perinuclear staining by IFA (pANCA— i.e., perinuclear ANCA). It is commonly seen in association with MPA (70% of patients) and EGPA (50% of patients), as well as in some patients with GPA and Goodpasture syndrome.

- Interpretation of the significance of the ANCA result must be made in association with the clinical picture. In a compatible clinical context, a positive cANCA result **combined with** a positive anti-PR3 assay result, or a positive pANCA result combined with a positive anti-MPO assay result, conveys more than 95% specificity for AAV.

- In AAV, positivity for both cANCA **and** pANCA in the same patient, or for anti-MPO **and** anti-PR3 in the same patient, is not expected. This finding should raise the hypothesis of an alternative diagnosis such as drug-induced vasculitis or cocaine or levamisole vasculopathy.

- ANCA positivity does not occur in PAN.

- Serial changes in ANCA, anti-PR3, or anti-MPO results do not correlate well with clinical remission or relapse in most patients, and thus must be viewed with consideration of the clinical appearance of the patient.

Anti-glomerular basement membrane (anti-GBM) antibodies: Anti-GBM antibodies are present in Goodpasture syndrome (anti-GBM disease) and in a minority of patients with AAV, usually MPO-ANCA. When both antibodies are present, initial presentation is that of

Goodpasture syndrome, with severe renal presentation. The natural history, however, is that of AAV with relapses; by contrast, Goodpasture syndrome usually does not recur.

EMG: This is useful in confirming myositis, neuropathy, and mononeuritis multiplex.

ECG: This may help detect myocardial ischemia, infarction, arrhythmia, and pericardial effusion.

Vascular imaging: This may help to identify medium- and large-artery involvement (e.g., PAN, TA, GCA). As conventional angiography is an invasive procedure, it is usually replaced by computed tomography angiography (CTA) or magnetic resonance angiography (MRA), although conventional angiography provides better imaging of medium-sized vessels (e.g., PAN).

Chest X-ray: This should be done in all patients with suspected systemic vasculitis. Note that findings may be normal in the presence of pulmonary hemorrhage.

Chest CT: Consider this in most patients with suspicion of systemic vasculitis, especially if hemoptysis is reported or there are concerns for pulmonary involvement.

Transthoracic echocardiogram: Use this according to clinical presentation. All EGPA patients should have an echocardiogram at baseline, as the finding of myocardial involvement may be of prognostic value.

Pulmonary function test: This is useful to screen for interstitial lung disease as a result of vasculitis (active disease, fibrosis) or treatment. It is also useful to screen for laryngotracheal stenosis. Very high diffusing capacity (DLCO) might indicate pulmonary hemorrhage.

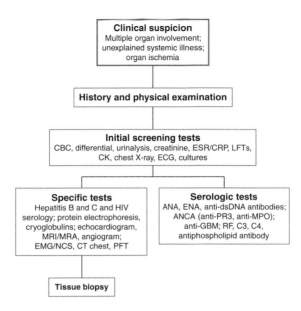

FIGURE 5a.2. Vasculitis diagnostic algorithm. Abbreviations: ANA, antinuclear antibody; ANCA, antineutrophil cytoplasmic antibody; anti-dsDNA, anti-double-stranded DNA; anti-GBM, anti-glomerular basement membrane; anti-MPO, antimyeloperoxidase; anti-PR3, anti-proteinase 3; ENA, extractable nuclear antigen; CK, creatine kinase; EMG, electromyography; LFTs, liver function tests; MRA, magnetic resonance angiography; NCS, nerve conduction study; PFT, pulmonary function test; RF, rheumatoid factor.

Figure 5a.2 presents a summary of the diagnostic approach to a patient with suspected vasculitis.

Pathological Findings

Figure 5a.3 shows a representation of the pathological findings in systemic vasculitides. Note that the individual vasculitis syndromes can be distinguished by size and type of vessel involvement, type of cell infiltration, and presence or absence of immune deposits or other characteristic features.

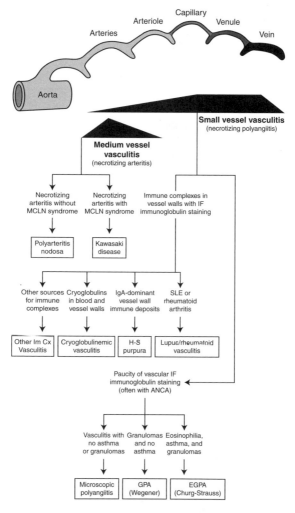

FIGURE 5a.3. Pathological findings in medium and small vessel vasculitis. Abbreviations: ANCA, antineutrophil cytoplasmic antibody; EPGA, eosinophilic granulomatosis with polyangiitis (previously known as Churg-Strauss syndrome); GPA, granulomatosis with polyangiitis (previously known as Wegener granulomatosis); H-S purpura, Henoch-Schönlein purpura; IF, immunofluorescence; Im Cx, immune complex; MCLS, mucocutaneous lymph node syndrome; SLE, systemic lupus erythematosus. Modified with permission from Jennette et al.[2]

Initial Therapy

- The treatment of systemic vasculitis is dependent on the specific diagnosis. Some conditions respond readily to relatively low doses of glucocorticoid therapy, some require higher doses, and others require more aggressive immune-modulating therapy to achieve a clinical remission. Several biologic agents have been studied in controlled trials and may be indicated under particular circumstances.

- Other factors may determine the therapy used, including: the severity of the illness, the particular organs affected, concomitant illnesses, and the ability of the patient to tolerate specific therapies. Consultation with a rheumatologist should always be sought when managing patients with vasculitis.

- Vasculitis identified as secondary to a known cause—such as infection, neoplasm, CTD, or medications or drugs—should be treated accordingly.

- In most cases, mortality in systemic vasculitides is the consequence of infectious complications and cardiovascular disease, not the vasculitis itself. Thus, prevention of, and active screening for, potential comorbidities should be part of standard treatment:
  - Avoid overimmunosuppression (this requires careful attention).
  - Pursue vaccinations (influenza, pneumococcal, zoster). Do this before immunosuppression, if possible.
  - Prescribe prophylactic antibiotics where appropriate (e.g., trimethoprim-sulfamethoxazole DS 3 times weekly while taking cyclophosphamide or other potent

immunosuppressive therapy to prevent *Pneumocystis jirovecii* infection).
- Pursue osteoporosis prevention.
- Manage cardiovascular risk factors.

CUTANEOUS LIMITED VASCULITIS

- Dapsone, colchicine, or glucocorticoids, orally in low dose or as a steroid ointment, may be effective in treating mild cutaneous vasculitic syndromes.
  - Low-dose glucocorticoids may also be useful for leukocytoclastic vasculitis associated with a drug reaction, infection, or malignancy.
  - For more important manifestations, moderate- to high-dose glucocorticoids may be required, in association with immunosuppressive agents such as methotrexate or azathioprine.
  - Leukocytoclastic vasculitis associated with hepatitis C is best treated with antiviral therapy such as pegylated interferon and ribavirin.
  - Protease inhibitors may have a role for the most severe manifestations of cryoglobulinemic vasculitis.

- Antihistamine drugs may provide symptomatic relief in patients with urticarial vasculitis, although they do not alter the disease course.

HENOCH-SCHÖNLEIN PURPURA

- HSP usually responds to glucocorticoids in children and adults.
- Patients can develop complications of glomerulonephritis or intra-abdominal complications, but these manifestations usually do not affect prognosis, which is generally good.
- Hypertension, declining renal function, significant proteinuria, or evidence of

mesenteric ischemia may indicate the need for additional immunosuppressive drugs such as cyclophosphamide.

GIANT CELL ARTERITIS AND TAKAYASU ARTERITIS

- A glucocorticoid (starting dose usually of 0.8–1 mg/kg/d prednisone equivalent) alone is very effective in the treatment of GCA. The dose is then reduced slowly over a 1- to 2-year period.
  - Relapses are frequent, however, and longer duration of treatment may be necessary.
  - ASA may decrease the risk of cerebral ischemic events and thus should be prescribed if not contraindicated by other medical conditions.

- A glucocorticoid is used as first-line treatment in TA, although relapses and disease progression are frequent despite continued therapy.
  - Small uncontrolled trials suggest benefit with concomitant use of systemic glucocorticoids and 1 of the following: methotrexate, azathioprine, tumour necrosis factor inhibitors, or tocilizumab.
  - Revascularization procedures by arterial bypass procedure or percutaneous endovascular interventions may be required for critical narrowing of arteries in TA.

GPA, MPA, AND EGPA

For disease that does not involve organs and is not life-threatening:

- **GPA:** Systemic glucocorticoids in combination with methotrexate may be an adequate option.
- **MPA and EGPA with a 5-factor score (FFS) of 0:** Glucocorticoids alone may be adequate.

FIVE-FACTOR SCORE (FFS)

The FFS is based on the identification of 5 prognostic markers:

1. CNS involvement
2. Severe GI disease
3. Proteinuria ≥ 1 g/d
4. Serum creatinine > 140 µmol/L
5. Cardiomyopathy

Each item counts for 1 point. A score of ≥ 1 predicts a higher mortality rate.

For disease that involves organs or is life-threatening (GPA, MPA, EGPA):

- High-dose systemic glucocorticoids (1 mg/kg/d prednisone equivalent, starting dose) in combination with cyclophosphamide should be prescribed for induction of remission.

- Cyclophosphamide may be given orally or as intermittent IV pulses, as both options are equivalent in terms of achieving remission. IV pulses may be associated with a higher rate of relapse.

- Remission is usually achieved within 3 to 6 months, at which time cyclophosphamide is switched to either methotrexate or azathioprine.

- Rituximab is an alternative to cyclophosphamide (GPA and MPA), especially for patients with relapsing disease, or at risk of toxicity or infertility.

- Steroids are usually weaned over a 6- to 18-month period.

POLYARTERITIS NODOSA

- **PAN with an FFS of 0:** This may be treated with glucocorticoids only.

- **PAN associated with hepatitis B infection:** Very good outcomes have been reported with a combination of a very short course of systemic glucocorticoids in association with plasmapheresis and antiviral therapy.

- More potent immunosuppressive treatment is reserved for patients with higher disease activity (e.g., FFS of 1 or higher, or organ or life-threatening disease).

KAWASAKI DISEASE

- Patients with KD receive high-dose salicylate therapy to reduce the incidence of coronary artery aneurysms.
- Patients often respond dramatically to IV gammaglobulin, especially when given within the first week of disease onset.

BEHÇET DISEASE

- Orogenital lesions are treated with topical application of glucocorticoid.
- Mucocutaneous manifestations and arthritis in BD may respond to the use of colchicine. Thalidomide may also be used for mucocutaneous features of the disease, although adverse events (neuropathy) are common. Thalidomide is contraindicated in pregnancy.
- Glucocorticoids are indicated for the treatment of BD, but this has not been reported in controlled studies. The combination of glucocorticoid and immunosuppressant therapy is used when vital organs are involved. Azathioprine, cyclophosphamide, and cyclosporine have been used. Encouraging results with tumour necrosis factor inhibitors have been reported in arthritic, ophthalmologic, CNS, GI, and refractory mucocutaneous manifestations.
- Anticoagulation therapy is controversial in cases of deep venous thrombosis and, thus, is not recommended. In BD, inflammation is at

the root of thrombotic complications. Hence, deep venous thrombosis is usually treated with immunosuppression.

GOODPASTURE SYNDROME

- The treatment of choice is plasmapheresis in combination with glucocorticoids and cyclophosphamide.
- Screening for ANCA should be performed, as the presence of these antibodies is associated with risk of relapse.

ACKNOWLEDGEMENT

Thanks to Dr. Avril Fitzgerald, University of Calgary, who developed this chapter for the first edition of the *Canadian Residents' Rheumatology Handbook*, 2005.

References

1. Jennette JC, Falk RJ, Bacon PA, et al. 2012 revised International Chapel Hill Consensus Conference Nomenclature of Vasculitides. *Arthritis Rheum.* 2013;65(1):1–11. http://dx.doi.org/10.1002/art.37715. Medline:23045170

2. Jennette JC, Thomas DB, Falk RJ. Microscopic polyangiitis (microscopic polyarteritis). *Semin Diagn Pathol.* 2001;18(1):3–13. Medline:11296991

Further Reading

Center for Disease Control. Kawasaki disease – New York. *MMWR Morb Mortal Wkly Rep.* 1980;29(6):61–3.

Hunder GG, Arend WP, Bloch DA, et al. The American College of Rheumatology 1990 criteria for the classification of vasculitis: Introduction. *Arthritis Rheum.* 1990; 33:1065–7 (see also pp. 1088 [polyarteritis nodosa], 1094 [Churg-Strauss syndrome], 1101 [Wegener granulomatosis], 1122 [giant cell arteritis], and 1129 [Takayasu]).

Jennette JC, Falk RJ. Small-vessel vasculitis. *N Engl J Med.* 1997;337(21):1512–23. http://dx.doi.org/10.1056/NEJM199711203372106. Medline:9366584

Kallenberg CG, Brouwer E, Weening JJ, et al. Antineutrophil cytoplasmic antibodies: current diagnostic and pathophysiological potential. *Kidney Int.* 1994;46(1):1–15. http://dx.doi.org/10.1038/ki.1994.239. Medline:7933826

Michel BA, Hunder GG, Bloch DA, et al. Hypersensitivity vasculitis and Henoch-Schönlein purpura: a comparison between the 2 disorders. *J Rheumatol.* 1992;19(5):721–8. Medline:1613701

The Patient Who Is Systemically Unwell

Is It a Connective Tissue Disease?

DR. STEPHANIE KEELING
DR. PAUL DAVIS
UNIVERSITY OF ALBERTA

KEY CONCEPTS

1. Multisystem connective tissue diseases (also called collagen vascular diseases) comprise a heterogeneous group of conditions that include: systemic lupus erythematosus (SLE); systemic sclerosis (scleroderma); mixed connective tissue disease (MCTD); polymyositis (PM) and dermatomyositis (DM); Sjögren syndrome; overlap syndromes; and undifferentiated connective tissue disease. Rheumatoid arthritis is sometimes included in this group.

2. These autoimmune diseases are generally characterized by sustained, systemic inflammation and a range of autoantibodies. (Scleroderma is an exception in that it may be inflammatory early in the disease process, but most disease manifestations are due to tissue fibrosis and/or vasculopathy.)

3. In all conditions, the disease may present insidiously (leading to delay in diagnosis) or acutely, constituting a rheumatologic emergency. Many manifestations are nonspecific and can consequently lead to confusion

in differential diagnosis. The pattern of organ system involvement may help define a specific diagnosis.

4. Early undifferentiated disease may manifest with common features such as arthritis, serositis, small vessel vasculitis, skin rash, myositis, and systemic manifestations of fever, weight loss, and fatigue. Nonspecific inflammatory markers (e.g., anemia, elevated ESR and CRP) and markers of autoreactivity (e.g., the presence of antinuclear antibody) may be seen (see chapter 10). Over time, the clinical syndrome of most patients evolves with a characteristic pattern and autoantibody profile.

5. Patients who show distinct features of 2 or more diseases may be characterized as having an overlap syndrome, and those with less specific features may be characterized as having undifferentiated connective tissue disease in the long term.

Overview of Connective Tissue Diseases

SYSTEMIC LUPUS ERYTHEMATOSUS (SLE)

- SLE is characterized by clinical features resulting from immune-mediated inflammation provoked by in-situ (e.g., glomerulonephritis) or circulating immune complexes (e.g., glomerulonephritis, vasculitis), or by direct antibody-mediated toxicity (e.g., autoimmune hemolytic anemia).

- Manifestations are protean and can involve almost every organ.

- Common presentations include a variety of skin rashes, arthritis, serositis, glomerulonephritis, and CNS involvement.

- SLE is associated with an increased risk for cardiovascular morbidity over time.

SYSTEMIC SCLEROSIS (SCLERODERMA)

- Systemic sclerosis is characterized by the deposition of abnormal and/or excessive collagen in the connective tissue of skin, gut, and lung, producing a picture of tissue fibrosis.

- An associated vasculopathy (noninflammatory structural and functional abnormalities) contributes to Raynaud phenomenon, pulmonary hypertension, and other clinical features of the disease.

- The limited form and diffuse form of systemic sclerosis are distinguished by the extent of skin involvement and a particular pattern of organ involvement.

POLYMYOSITIS (PM) AND DERMATOMYOSITIS (DM)

- These inflammatory disorders of skeletal muscle occur with or without skin involvement.

- Each has characteristic clinical features, histopathological characteristics, and immune markers (see chapter 3).

- Patients may have associated features of arthritis and vasculopathy or vasculitis.

SJÖGREN SYNDROME

- Sjögren syndrome is a cell-mediated autoimmune disorder of exocrine glands.

- Clinical features can usually be predicted on the basis of reduced volume and/or increased viscosity of exocrine secretions.

- The most common manifestations are keratoconjunctivitis sicca (dry eyes) and xerostomia (dry mouth).

- Many other inflammatory organ manifestations are possible.

- The disease can exist on its own (primary) or occur in association with another rheumatic disease such as rheumatoid arthritis (secondary).

Collagen vascular

MIXED CONNECTIVE TISSUE DISEASE (MCTD)

- This disease is characterized by the presence of elements of SLE, inflammatory myositis, and scleroderma.

- It is also characterized by a particular autoantibody profile: antiribonucleoprotein (anti-RNP).

- Although similar to an overlap syndrome, MCTD is considered a distinct clinical entity. Common features include sclerodactyly, Raynaud phenomenon, and myositis.

History

A carefully documented history of disease manifestations over time is important to making a diagnosis.

PATIENT DEMOGRAPHICS

These conditions frequently present in young or middle-aged females, although none of them are age and sex specific. Juvenile and elderly forms of these diseases exist, but are less common.

KEY QUESTIONS

These questions seek to establish whether the patient:

- has organ involvement that is typical for connective tissue disease

- presents with a pattern of organ involvement characteristic of a particular entity

- has a presentation that can be explained by another diagnosis (e.g., infection, vasculitis, endocrinopathy, etc.)

- has critical organ involvement requiring urgent attention (e.g., CNS, renal, hematologic, or vascular involvement)

1. Do you have constitutional symptoms?

Weight loss, fatigue, anorexia, and low-grade fever are common but nonspecific.

2. Do you have arthralgias or arthritis?

- A history in keeping with inflammatory arthritis (see chapter 2) will provide stronger objective evidence for a connective tissue disease.
- Myalgia may also be an early feature of several diseases.

3. Do you have Raynaud phenomenon?

- The diagnosis of Raynaud phenomenon requires episodic, well-demarcated blanching of the digits, and a history or observation of pallor. Some patients may only have acrocyanosis (see chapter 4).
- With a positive history, inquire about secondary effects (i.e., digital pits, ulcers, and loss of digital pulp).

4. Is there mucocutaneous involvement?

- Various skin rashes are seen in SLE.
- Classic skin rashes are part of DM (see chapter 3).
- Skin thickening or tightening is a feature of systemic sclerosis. It may begin with "puffy" hands, which is also a feature of MCTD.
- Alopecia is seen in lupus: ask about excessive hairs (more than 20) on the pillow in the morning.
- Oral ulcers may be painful or painless.

5. Is there muscle weakness?

Proximal muscle weakness is a feature of PM/DM, but it may also develop in MCTD or SLE.

6. Are there sicca symptoms?

- Dry eyes are characterized by grittiness, lids sticking in the morning, burning pain, and redness. The patient may have a thick discharge.
- Dry mouth is characterized by difficulty eating without liquids, water needed at the bedside, and increased dental caries. Ask: "Can you chew and swallow a soda cracker without water?"

Collagen vascular

7. Is there serositis?

- Pleuritic chest pain could represent pleuritis or pericarditis. A pulmonary embolism in a patient with SLE and antiphospholipid antibodies may also present this way.

- Abdominal serositis may present as nonspecific abdominal pain.

8. Are there any cardiorespiratory problems?

Some patients may have early manifestations of interstitial lung disease.

9. Is there any history of blood clots or miscarriages?

Patients with lupus may have associated antiphospholipid antibodies with the attendant clinical manifestations.

10. Is there any other medical history?

- Taking a careful medical history is important, as previous medical conditions or events may not have been recognized for their significance (e.g., a history of "idiopathic" thrombocytopenic purpura may have greater significance in the face of a possible connective tissue disease diagnosis).

- A careful review of past medical records and investigations is often helpful.

11. Is there a family history of autoimmune or rheumatic diseases?

Family history can sometimes assist in making the clinical diagnosis, but diagnosis should not rely on family history.

Physical Examination

General approach:

- The pattern of organ system involvement over time may help with a specific diagnosis.

- The specific features of the organ system involved must be determined and documented by a physician for accurate disease diagnosis.
- It is important to determine whether there are any clinical features requiring urgent attention.
- The distribution of organ involvement by disease is summarized in Table 5b.1.

Vital signs: Look for tachycardia (pericarditis, myocarditis, anemia, etc.), tachypnea, fever, hypertension (glomerulonephritis or other renal involvement).

Head and neck (including scalp): Look for alopecia, ocular inflammation (e.g., scleritis), oral and nasal ulcerations, malar rash, telangiectasia, lymphadenopathy.

Chest: Check for crackles (interstitial lung disease), decreased air entry or rubs (pleural effusions, pleuritis).

Cardiovascular exam: Check for rubs, signs of pulmonary hypertension, congestive heart failure, new murmurs (endocarditis: bacterial or Libman-Sacks).

Musculoskeletal exam: Look for swollen or tender joints (synovitis), muscle weakness (proximal muscle for inflammatory myositis).

Skin:

- Look for rashes, purpura, nodules.
- Examine fingertips for pits, periungual erythema, telangiectasia, hemorrhages, or infarcts, as well as sclerodactyly (thickening and tightening of skin).

Neurologic exam: Check for focal deficits, encephalopathy, psychosis, symptoms of peripheral neuropathy or mononeuritis multiplex.

Collagen vascular

TABLE 5b.1. Common clinical features of connective tissue diseases by organ system

Organ system	Lupus	Scleroderma	Polymyositis/dermatomyositis	Sjögren syndrome
Locomotor	Nonerosive synovitis Avascular necrosis Jaccoud arthropathy	Puffy, shiny hands (early) Joint (tendon) contractures, tendon friction rubs	Muscle wasting, weakness, and tenderness Arthritis possible in some DM presentations	Arthralgia/arthritis
Mucocutaneous	Discoid lupus erythematosus Malar (butterfly) rash Alopecia Photosensitivity Oral ulcers Conjunctivitis	Digital pits Sclerodactyly Scleroderma Calcinosis Telangiectasia	Gottron papules Heliotrope rash Periungual vasculitis V-sign Shawl sign	Dry mucous membranes: • Xerophthalmia • Xerostomia, pulmonary and genital secretions
Renal	Glomerulonephritis Nephrotic/nephritic syndrome Acute renal failure (AKI)	Acute renal failure (AKI) and/or hypertensive emergency: • Scleroderma renal crisis (see chapter 15: can be normotensive)		Distal renal tubular acidosis (type 4)

(Continued)

TABLE 5b.1. (Continued)

Organ system	Lupus	Scleroderma	Polymyositis/dermatomyositis	Sjögren syndrome
CNS	Seizure disorder	Seizures in setting of hypertensive crisis	Proximal muscle weakness (should be distinguished from motor neuron disease, polyradiculopathy, myasthenia gravis, etc.)	MS-like syndrome
	Psychiatric disorders			Peripheral neuropathy
	Migraine, acute stroke (secondary to antiphospholipid antibody syndrome)			
	Peripheral neuropathy			
Cardiovascular	Raynaud phenomenon	Raynaud phenomenon, pulmonary hypertension	Cardiomyopathy	
	Pericarditis	Vasculopathy, restrictive cardiomyopathy (secondary to ischemia)		
	Endocarditis (Libman Sacks endocarditis), premature coronary artery disease, secondary hypertension			
	Vascular thrombosis (antiphospholipid antibody syndrome)			
Pulmonary	Pleuritis and effusion	Pulmonary fibrosis	Interstitial lung disease (think anti-synthetase syndrome)	Interstitial lung disease
	Pneumonitis	Pulmonary hypertension		
	Pulmonary hemorrhage			
	Shrinking lung syndrome			
	Pulmonary embolus (secondary to antiphospholipid syndrome)			

Collagen vascular

(Continued)

TABLE 5b.1. (Continued)

Organ system	Lupus	Scleroderma	Polymyositis/dermatomyositis	Sjögren syndrome
GI	Peritonitis Small bowel vasculitis Autoimmune hepatitis (rare)	Dysphagia, reflux Small bowel dysmotility and large bowel pseudo-obstruction	Dysphagia due to involvement of esophageal musculature	
Hematologic	Cytopenias Antiphospholipid antibody syndrome	Anemia (microangiopathic hemolytic) in context of renal crisis		Lymphoma

Abbreviations: AKI, acute kidney injury; DM, dermatomyositis; MS, multiple sclerosis.

Additional notes:

- Manifestations of disease may only appear over time.
- Sjögren syndrome can be associated with other rheumatologic disorders (e.g., secondary).
- Antiphospholipid antibody syndrome can occur as a primary disorder or in association with other connective tissue disease, most notably SLE.
- Myositis may be associated with malignancies.

Key Laboratory Investigations

Laboratory testing should be guided by the history and examination, and investigations should first address specific "target organs" involved clinically before autoimmune serological analysis is ordered. Few investigations are specific to the underlying condition, with the exception of some nuclear autoantibodies. Some tests are as important for monitoring drug therapy toxicity as they are for disease treatment.

CBC, platelet count, and differential: These assess cytopenias (SLE), eosinophilia (various connective tissue diseases with or without vasculitis); they also monitor for medication toxicity.

Creatinine, urea, electrolytes: These identify features of azotemia in acute or chronic renal failure (SLE, scleroderma, Sjögren syndrome).

Urinalysis: This identifies protein, blood, and casts as features of membranous or proliferative glomerulonephritis (SLE).

Muscle enzymes: Muscle enzymes are a manifestation of myositis (PM, lupus).

Antibodies to specific nuclear antigens (see also chapter 10):

ANA is nonspecific and can be present in any connective tissue disease (as well as in normal and many other conditions).

Anti-Sm, anti-double-stranded DNA is specific to SLE.

Anti-Ro/La is associated with Sjögren syndrome and also seen in SLE.

Anti-RNP is associated with MCTD, but can be seen in conjunction with other extractable nuclear antigens in SLE.

Anti-Jo-1 is associated with antisynthetase syndrome in myositis (interstitial lung disease, rheumatoid-arthritis-like polyarthritis, "mechanic's hands").

Anti-Scl-70 and anticentromere antibody are associated with diffuse and limited scleroderma, respectively.

Double-stranded DNA antibodies (anti-dsDNA): This is positive in a subset of SLE patients. It may or may not parallel (it may or may not be "concordant" with) disease activity in SLE patients (e.g., nephritis, pulmonary hemorrhage). It can be positive in overlap patients with features of SLE and other connective tissue diseases.

Complement levels: These are reduced with complement activation due to immune complex formation (SLE). They might be elevated as an acute phase reactant in myositis and vasculitis.

ECG: This can provide evidence of pericarditis (SLE), cardiomyopathy (myositis), ischemia (especially in long-standing disease).

Chest X-ray: This can identify features of pleuritis with pleural effusion (SLE), pulmonary fibrosis, (scleroderma, DM).

Echocardiogram: This can identify pulmonary hypertension (scleroderma), pericardial effusion (SLE).

Tissue biopsy: Collect biopsy specimens as warranted: renal (SLE, occasionally for scleroderma), muscle (PM/DM), minor salivary (labial) gland (Sjögren syndrome), skin (SLE, DM).

Other tests: The following tests have low value for distinguishing among connective tissue diseases: liver function tests, serum urate, ESR, CRP, rheumatoid factor, ANA.

Treatment Options

- The diversity and complexity of organ-system involvement dictates that each case be treated individually.
- The treatment approach includes monotherapy or combination therapy to achieve disease remission while evaluating the risk-benefit ratio of the medication(s).
- Drug-drug interaction and drug side effects can significantly add to the complexity of disease management.
- The evolution of the disease and its manifestations over time will necessitate regular review of pharmacotherapy.
- It is essential to appropriately monitor all drugs for side effects over time and to institute prophylaxis where appropriate (e.g., for glucocorticoid-induced osteoporosis).
- Therapies are usually instituted for longer rather than shorter periods to maintain low disease activity or a disease remission state.
- The long-term prognosis may be influenced by evolving features of the disease itself, long-term complications of inflammatory disease (e.g., premature coronary artery disease in SLE), or side effects of long-term drug therapy (infection, osteoporosis, avascular necrosis). It is important

Collagen vascular

to monitor closely and to institute preemptive therapy or prophylaxis where appropriate.

GENERAL APPROACH TO THERAPY
This section lists therapies have proven value in certain clinical situations.

Topical preparations
Glucocorticoid creams are of value in the management of cutaneous manifestations of lupus and DM.

- Use only low-potency glucocorticoids on the face.
- Consider topical calcineurin inhibitors.
- Sunscreen is an important addition to prevent skin flares and drug-related photodermatitis.
- Artificial tears and other ophthalmologic lubricants are helpful for keratoconjunctivitis sicca.
- Oral lubricants are available for xerostomia (dry mouth). Chewing sugarless gum or candies can stimulate salivary flow. Meticulous dental care is essential.

Nonsteroidal anti-inflammatory drugs (NSAIDs) and analgesics
- NSAIDs and analgesics are useful for nonspecific symptomatic relief of musculoskeletal symptoms and mild pericarditis.
- Care must be given to monitor BP, renal function, and GI ulcer risk (see chapter 12).

Antimalarials
- Antimalarial drugs are of particular value in multiple lupus manifestations, including skin and joint disease, and are useful in DM skin disease.
- They are proven to reduce future flares of SLE (renal and nonrenal) and are useful and safe in

pregnancy to control disease. Most patients with lupus should be taking an antimalarial drug.

- They are often used in combination with other immunosuppressants.
- Regular ophthalmologic monitoring is required.

Glucocorticoids (oral and parenteral)

- Glucocorticoids are often used as first-line therapy because of their quick onset of action for many of the inflammatory manifestations of the various diseases, including arthritis, pleuritis, pericarditis, and glomerulonephritis or myositis.
- They are valuable as a single agent or in combination with immunosuppressives for nephritis or other severe disease manifestations.
- **Avoid the "shotgun" approach of introducing steroids before every effort has been made to establish the diagnosis. In a patient with organ- or life-threatening disease, steroids may need to be introduced while investigations are ongoing** (see also chapter 12).

Immunosuppressives

- Azathioprine (Imuran) and methotrexate, in combination with steroids, are of value in many of these diseases as part of initial therapy or for a "steroid-sparing" effect (e.g., nonrenal SLE, active myositis).
- Mycophenolate mofetil (Cellcept) or mycophenolic acid (Myfortic) are:
  - equivalent to cyclophosphamide for induction of class 3 and class 4 glomerulonephritis (proliferative glomerulonephritis) in lupus
  - beneficial for nonrenal lupus and DM
  - preferred for young patients and those of Afro-Caribbean and Hispanic descent

Collagen vascular

- Cyclophosphamide as a single agent or in combination with steroids:
  - is of value for proliferative glomerulonephritis (particularly for postmenopausal women and older men of European descent)
  - is also used for pulmonary hemorrhage, CNS lupus
  - is used in life-threatening myositis (e.g., respiratory failure)
  - can suppress the parenchymal pulmonary manifestations of systemic sclerosis
  - is available via several regimens
- Biologic therapies can be of value:
  - Rituximab (Rituxan) may be beneficial for refractory SLE and myositis when other first-line agents are not working.
  - Belimumab (Benlysta) is beneficial for seropositive SLE (positive ANA and/or positive anti-dsDNA) with moderate to severe disease, but trials excluded active lupus nephritis or CNS lupus patients.
  - Biologic therapies are beneficial for skin and joint manifestations of lupus.
  - They may allow for glucocorticoids to be tapered.

SPECIAL SITUATIONS

Antiphospholipid syndrome (primary or secondary)
Treat this syndrome for anticoagulation as warranted.

Raynaud phenomenon (primary or secondary)
See chapter 4.

Pulmonary hypertension (systemic sclerosis)
Treat pulmonary hypertension with IV epoprostenol or bosentan (Tracleer) as warranted.

Malignant hypertension (systemic sclerosis)
Treat malignant hypertension with angiotensin-

converting enzyme inhibitors as warranted (see chapter 16).

Xerophthalmia/xerostomia (Sjögren syndrome)

Treat this syndrome with pilocarpine (Salogen).

Further Reading

Given the breadth of material covered in this chapter, specific references are not provided. A general rheumatology textbook would be a good starting point for more in-depth reading about specific conditions. A good overview of conditions discussed in this chapter can be found in the following reference:

Klippel JH, Stone JH, Crofford LJ, et al, editors. Primer on the rheumatic diseases. 13th ed. New York: Springer; 2008. http://dx.doi.org/10.1007/978-0-387-68566-3.

Collagen vascular

6

Diffuse Musculoskeletal Pain and the Diagnosis of Fibromyalgia

DR. MARY-ANN FITZCHARLES
MCGILL UNIVERSITY

Fibromyalgia (FM) is a polysymptomatic condition with a pivotal symptom of diffuse body pain, but with other associated symptoms such as sleep disturbance, fatigue, cognitive dysfunction, mood disorder, and various somatic symptoms.[1] Symptoms may be present to a variable degree in individual patients and may vary over time. Although the exact cause of FM is unknown, the abnormality is currently believed to be centred in the nervous system and represents a dysregulation of pain-processing mechanisms.

There is no clinical biomarker or objective abnormality to aid the clinician in confirming the diagnosis. FM may present as a stand-alone diagnosis in an individual, or may occur in conjunction with another rheumatic disease such as rheumatoid arthritis (RA), systemic lupus erythematosus, and others. The recognition of FM as a comorbid condition with other rheumatic diseases is important, as treatments can be directed toward FM if the primary disease is controlled. Guidelines for the diagnosis, management, and follow-up of patients with FM have been recently developed for Canada.[2]

KEY CONCEPTS
1. Widespread musculoskeletal pain is a common problem.
2. There is a wide differential diagnosis for this problem, including: rheumatic disease; neurologic conditions; endocrine disorders; somatization and other mental health disorders; and medication side effects. A careful history and physical examination are essential.
3. FM is common and can be positively diagnosed after a full clinical evaluation and simple blood testing. Consider FM as the cause of widespread pain in a middle-aged woman who has had a gradual onset of pain and associated somatic symptoms.

History

PATIENT DEMOGRAPHICS
FM has been estimated to affect between 2% and 4% of the adult population in Canada. Although most commonly recognized in women in the middle years of life, FM may affect children, men, and the elderly.

KEY QUESTIONS

1. Is the pain chronic?
- Pain must have been present for at least 3 months to be classified as chronic.
- Pain present for 3 or more months may be due to an intercurrent self-limited illness (e.g., a viral illness).

2. Is the pain generalized?
- Some patients with FM report pain from the top of the head to the soles of the feet.
- For some, pain moves from site to site in a waxing-and-waning pattern, with variable intensity and location.

- Some patients identify a specific focus area of pain, but with an associated generalized pain.
- If pain is localized to specific joints or areas, consider whether there is a pattern that fits with inflammatory arthritis (possibly with secondary FM), multiple regional problems (e.g., tendinitis in shoulder and bursitis in hip), or another disorder.

3. What characterizes the pain?

- The pain quality in FM is an aching muscle pain, with patients commonly saying "I feel as if I have run a marathon." About one-third of patients describe pain that has neuropathic qualities (e.g., burning or tingling).
- Some patients have a subjective feeling of joint swelling and even total-body stiffness, although true joint swelling does not occur in FM.

4. Was the onset of pain gradual or acute?

- FM generally has a gradual and insidious onset, with many patients reporting some degree of aches and pains over many years, with increased severity prompting consultation.
- A triggering event is reported in up to 30% of patients with FM (e.g., following a physical illness such as a viral infection or following psychological or physical trauma in the absence of a tissue lesion to explain the pain).[3]
  - If a traumatic event has preceded the onset of FM, there should be a continuum in time without hiatus before causation can be attributed to that event.
- The preceding physical and mental health status must be reviewed, as there may have been past indications of chronic pain.
- Question the diagnosis of FM if the onset is abrupt: consider a drug-induced syndrome,

an acute process related to an infectious or neoplastic process, or polymyalgia rheumatica (PMR) in elderly patients.

5. What factors make the pain better or worse?

- Symptoms of FM may fluctuate spontaneously or be aggravated by barometric pressure changes, emotional stress and poor sleep, and physical activity (for one-third of patients).

- Symptoms may be relieved by a hot bath, relaxation, meditation, massage, or exercise.

- If FM is occurring concomitantly with a rheumatic disease such as RA, a flare of the inflammatory disease can aggravate FM features.

6. Are there any constitutional symptoms?

- Prominent constitutional features (i.e., fever, sweats, anorexia, weight loss) might indicate an underlying inflammatory or neoplastic disease, or an endocrinopathy.

- In the absence of definite constitutional features, low energy can be a feature of FM. Fatigue occurs for over 90% of patients with FM. It is often severe and may be more marked than in patients with inflammatory rheumatic diseases. Patients with FM will often just manage to complete their responsibilities and then go to bed very early in evening, or nap on the weekends or during the day in off-work hours.

- Weight gain is more typical of FM than weight loss.

7. Are there other somatic symptoms along with the generalized pain?

- FM is a polysymptomatic condition and other associated symptoms such as sleep disturbance, fatigue, cognitive dysfunction, mood disorder, and various somatic symptoms are associated with the chronic pain.

Widespread pain

- Given the range of symptoms found in patients with FM, it is important to ask questions carefully to determine whether there is an underlying rheumatic, neurologic, endocrine, or neoplastic disorder.

- Is there any joint swelling or morning stiffness suggestive of inflammatory arthritis? Is there any objective weakness (e.g., trouble climbing stairs or getting out of a chair) that is compatible with myositis? Are there any features compatible with a connective tissue disease (e.g., skin rash, alopecia, mucosal ulcers, dry eyes or mouth, serositis, peripheral edema, skin thickening, Raynaud phenomenon, etc.)? Is there any history of long-standing back stiffness, uveitis, or psoriasis, as with seronegative spondylarthritis, in which widespread pain may arise from enthesitis?

- Are there any neurologic symptoms (e.g., numbness, tingling, objective weakness, difficulty with speech or vision, etc.)?

- Is there bony pain or night pain suggestive of a neoplastic process such as myeloma?

- Symptoms associated with FM should be considered. Cognitive dysfunction is common, with difficulty concentrating (e.g., when reading a book, multitasking, remembering shopping lists). This has been termed "fibro fog." Mood disorder, including depression and anxiety, occurs for over half of patients and affects coping and motivation. Patients may have had mood disorder before the onset of FM, and the continuous symptoms may cause an exacerbation of poor mood.

- Body stiffness is present in FM, but is less severe than for patients with a rheumatic condition such as PMR or RA. Reported disability can be striking and appear out of proportion to almost-normal physical examination.

- Other somatic symptoms in FM include chronic headaches, irritable bowel syndrome, interstitial cystitis, and temporomandibular pain, among others.

8. What is your sleep like?

- Sleep is frequently disturbed in patients with FM, who say that they "just cannot sleep peacefully." FM patients seldom wake because of pain; rather, they wake for other reasons and then are conscious of pain.

- Sleep disturbance in FM usually consists of frequent awakening, prolonged periods of getting back to sleep, or awakening in the mornings exhausted.

- Patients with FM often spend prolonged periods in bed hoping to get restful sleep. This is in contrast, for example, to patients who have inflammatory spondylarthritis, who awaken in the second half of the night with pain and stiffness and who prefer staying active to being in bed.

9. How is your mood?

- Consider whether there is an underlying mental health issue and explore any psychosocial factors that might be relevant.

- Mood disorder, including depression and anxiety, occurs for over half of patients and impacts coping and motivation.

- Patients may have had mood disorder before the onset of FM, and the continuous symptoms may cause an exacerbation of poor mood.

10. Are there any previous health or mental health issues?

- Explore the history of previous pain disorders such as chronic headaches, prolonged recovery from acute back events, or previous mood disorder.

- A previous eating disorder or substance abuse may indicate evolution of a psychophysical illness.

- A preexisting diagnosis of a connective tissue disease may be associated with concomitant (secondary) FM.

11. What medications are you taking?

- Are there any new medications? Some drugs can be associated with musculoskeletal pain syndromes (e.g., statins, bisphosphonates, aromatase inhibitors).

- Although chemotherapy causes peripheral neuropathy, some patients may develop a more diffuse pain syndrome, especially if there was a background of FM.

12. Is there a family history of rheumatic disease? Is there a history of FM?

- A family history of chronic illness, disablement, and psychosocial disadvantage may be present for some FM patients.

- Patients often report that a mother or sibling has had similar symptoms, but without a definite diagnosis.

13. Have there been previous investigations?

- Patients with FM have commonly had symptoms for many years, and often have already had extensive laboratory and radiographic investigations.

- Test results are normal in FM. X-rays may show changes in keeping with the patient's age, especially for the spine.

14. What treatments have been tried?

- Most patients with FM will already have tried analgesic treatments, either self-administered with over-the-counter preparations or by prescription.
- Use of naturopathic, homeopathic, and other complementary products is prevalent in FM patients. There is currently insufficient evidence to support the use of any single product.

15. What is your functional capacity?

- Patients with FM can often be as disabled as those with underlying rheumatic or neurologic disease.
- Asking about the duration and acuity of symptoms may be helpful.

Physical Examination

Vitals: These will be normal in FM. Be alert to changes that indicate underlying disease (e.g., tachycardia due to hyperthyroidism).

Head and neck, chest, cardiovascular system, abdomen, and skin: Perform a screening examination to look for evidence of underlying disease.

Neurologic exam:

- There is no objective weakness in FM. Patients with FM may report subjective weakness, but with normal muscle strength on testing or inconsistent findings of weakness.
- Patients with FM may have dysesthesia (unpleasant sensations associated with touch), allodynia (pain with nonpainful stimuli), and generalized muscle tenderness to palpation. Expression of pain or pain behaviours may be present, but should not imply faking of symptoms.

Musculoskeletal exam: There should be no evidence of enthesitis, active synovitis in the joints, or restriction of spinal mobility in a patient with primary FM. The tender point examination is no longer a required defining feature of FM, in line with the 2010 American College of Rheumatology diagnostic criteria.[4]

Key Laboratory Investigations

- If FM is suspected, order a laboratory screen:
  - Include CBC, creatinine, urinalysis, liver enzymes, CK, calcium, thyroid-stimulating hormone (TSH).
  - Consider ESR and CRP, although these tests are insensitive and nonspecific.
  - Consider protein electrophoresis to screen for myeloma if appropriate.
- Any additional tests should be driven by findings on history or examination that suggest another underlying diagnosis.
- Routine blood work should be normal in FM.
- Avoid testing for antinuclear antibody unless other features support the diagnosis of a connective tissue disease. A low-positive titre can be seen in healthy individuals and the FM population (and should be considered as not clinically significant).
- Further immunological testing should be done only on clinical suspicion of connective tissue disease.
- Radiology imaging should be done only if there is a clinical impression of a condition such as inflammatory spondylarthritis or inflammatory arthritis.
- Electromyography in patients with FM is normal, even in the setting of mild neurologic symptoms. These studies should not be routinely requested unless there is a reasonable clinical suspicion of a true neurologic or myopathic process.

- Biopsy is not indicated if FM is a reasonable clinical diagnosis. Biopsy would only be done to confirm a clinical diagnosis of giant cell arteritis, myositis, myopathy, etc.

Differential Diagnosis

Conditions other than FM may present with features of generalized musculoskeletal pain.

Inflammatory rheumatic diseases

- Early RA and some connective tissue diseases present with generalized musculoskeletal pain.
- Consider polymyalgia rheumatica (PMR) in individuals over age 50 with more defined onset. Patients will often have sleep disruption due to pain. Pain and stiffness are prominent in the morning and after inactivity. There may be constitutional symptoms. Inflammatory markers (ESR, CRP) will be elevated.
- Consider inflammatory myositis when the clinical course is characterized by objective weakness more than pain. Individuals have difficulty rising from a chair, climbing stairs, and getting up from lying. They may have associated skin manifestations of dermatomyositis (see chapter 3).
- Consider systemic vasculitis in patients with prominent constitutional features, and calf and leg pain or claudication-like symptoms.

Viral syndromes

- Influenza can present with calf and leg pain and possibly an elevated CK.
- Consider enteroviruses (e.g., group B coxsackie virus, especially B5 and B6).
- Consider other viral causes (e.g., hepatitis B, rubella, herpes virus, respiratory syncytial virus, HIV).

Widespread pain

Drug-induced musculoskeletal syndromes

- Statins produce myalgias in 6% to 14% of patients. Other medications can inhibit statin metabolism, including itraconazole, cyclosporine, and erythromycin, as can electrolyte disturbances, infection, trauma, and hypoxia.

- Aromatase inhibitors, bisphosphonates, certain chemotherapy agents, proton pump inhibitors, quinolone antibiotics, steroids, colchicine, and other drugs can be associated with musculoskeletal pain.

Endocrinopathies

Consider hypothyroidism, hyperparathyroidism, Cushing syndrome.

Neurologic conditions

Consider multiple sclerosis, neuropathies, others.

Paraneoplastic phenomenon

Psychiatric disease

Consider depression, somatic symptom disorder, borderline personality disorders, drug-seeking behaviours.

Diagnosis of FM

- FM should be positively diagnosed after a full clinical evaluation and simple blood testing. It is no longer a diagnosis of exclusion.

- The criteria for the diagnosis of FM were revised by the American College of Rheumatology in 2010. Note that these criteria were developed to identify homogenous patient cohorts for the purpose of study and should not be used to diagnose individual patients.

  - The reason for not using the criteria is the variability of symptoms over time, with a single patient fulfilling or not fulfilling criteria at any particular time point.

- It is therefore important to conceptualize FM as a composite of subjective symptoms leading to a total global suffering.
- Individual personal psychosocial characteristics may also influence the expression of symptom severity.
- Those with an important mood disorder, such as depression or anxiety, or a catastrophizing or passive dependent personality, are likely to report more severe and resistant subjective symptoms.

Initial Therapy

- FM presents a challenge to the clinician:
  - Symptoms are heterogeneous and vary within and among patients.
  - Patients are generally perceived to be challenging, time-consuming, and complex to manage.
  - No clinical finding or biomarker confirms the diagnosis.
  - Treatments to date generally give only modest relief.
  - A societal culture of disablement due to this condition has evolved over the last 2 decades.

- Ideal management requires active patient participation in health-related practices.
- The essence of current evidence is that there is no "gold standard" of treatment, with responses mostly modest at best.
- Public education and social marketing will help demystify FM and promote health.

NONPHARMACOLOGIC STRATEGIES

- It is imperative that nonpharmacologic strategies are a component of management for every patient with FM.

Widespread pain

- Patients should be encouraged to develop a strong internal locus of control that promotes self-efficacy, coping skills, and good lifelong health-related habits; and that allows them to pursue as normal a life pattern as possible and, especially, to maintain routine. Retention in the workforce should be strongly encouraged.

- Regular physical activity should form the cornerstone of treatment of all patients and is strongly recommended by the 2012 Canadian FM guidelines.
  - Physical activity may take the form of an aerobic, strengthening, water, home-based, or group program, depending on availability for individual patients.
  - To facilitate adherence, engage the patient in making choices about activities.

- Instruction in sleep hygiene should be given to all patients before recourse to tranquillizing medications. Simple strategies such as regular sleeping habits, limited time recumbent in bed, avoiding excessive caffeine, and wind-down time before sleep are effective.

- Physical modalities such as heat may be beneficial, but patients should be discouraged from using physical aids that can promote the sickness role. Although many patients with FM are using various complementary and alternative medicines, in the absence of evidence, none can be recommended.

- Although multidisciplinary care is ideal, it is not available to all.
  - Access to a health care team member, especially a nurse who is knowledgeable about FM and can provide support and encouragement, may help to develop coping strategies.

- Participation in community activities such as exercise groups, support networks, and public education forums may be an effective substitute for multidisciplinary care.
- Education and active participation are key to effective self-management, rather than prolonged attendance at a specific program.

PHARMACOLOGIC OPTIONS

Drug treatments may be helpful for some patients, but they must be assessed for benefits and side effects, and should not be continued indefinitely unless the benefit clearly persists.

Many drug side effects mimic symptoms of FM:

- Fatigue may be aggravated by gabapentinoids, antidepressants, or analgesics.
- Depression may be exacerbated by opioids and cannabinoids.
- GI symptoms may be affected by nonsteroidal anti-inflammatory drugs, opioids, and antidepressants.
- Sleep disturbance may be aggravated by opioids and antidepressants.

Symptom-based management is a rational approach, with drugs that impact more than 1 symptom adding an advantage. Consider combinations of treatments and using lower doses than reported in drug studies.

The following list describes drug-treatment options.

Simple analgesics
- Opioid analgesics should be strongly discouraged or used only with extreme caution.
- In the absence of a formal study of opioids in FM, and with evidence for serious personal and

Widespread pain

societal adverse effects, any use of opioids should be strictly limited and monitored. Tramadol, an agent with weak opioid agonist activity as well as serotonin effects, has shown some benefit in FM, and generally has less serious adverse effects than strong opioid agents.

Tricyclic antidepressants (TCAs)

- Low-dose TCA medications such as amitriptyline have had a reported good effect for about one-third of patients. Use is limited by side effects of dry mouth, excessive daytime sleepiness, and weight gain.
- These agents may work by both optimizing sleep patterns and minimizing pain.
- Low doses in the early evening may be tried.

Selective serotonin reuptake inhibitors (SSRIs) and serotonin-norepinephrine reuptake inhibitors (SNRIs)

- Meta-analyses report that SSRIs and SNRIs may help some patients. However, outside these drugs' primary use for mood disorder, their effect is generally only modest.

Anticonvulsants such as gabapentinoids

- Gabapentinoids may have an effect on peripheral sensitization. They also promote good sleep architecture and reduction of anxiety.
- Use of these agents is limited by adverse cognitive effects and also weight gain.

Cyclobenzaprine

- This is a muscle relaxant structurally similar to TCA. It may be helpful for relief during a flare of symptoms.

Other agents

- Dopaminergic agents, sleep modifiers, synthetic cannabinoids, and atypical antipsychotic agents have been examined in small studies, but with none showing an outstanding effect.

- Consider these on a case-by-case basis.

References

1. Mease P, Arnold LM, Choy EH, et al; OMERACT Fibromyalgia Working Group. Fibromyalgia syndrome module at OMERACT 9: domain construct. *J Rheumatol.* 2009;36(10):2318–29. http://dx.doi.org/10.3899/jrheum.090367. Medline:19820221

2. Fitzcharles MA, Ste-Marie PA, Goldenberg DL, et al; National Fibromyalgia Guideline Advisory Panel. 2012 Canadian Guidelines for the diagnosis and management of fibromyalgia syndrome: executive summary. *Pain Res Manag.* 2013;18(3):119–26. Medline:23748251

3. Greenfield S, Fitzcharles MA, Esdaile JM. Reactive fibromyalgia syndrome. *Arthritis Rheum.* 1992;35(6):678–81. http://dx.doi.org/10.1002/art.1780350612. Medline:1599521

4. Wolfe F, Clauw DJ, Fitzcharles MA, et al. The American College of Rheumatology preliminary diagnostic criteria for fibromyalgia and measurement of symptom severity. *Arthritis Care Res (Hoboken).* 2010;62(5):600–10. http://dx.doi.org/10.1002/acr.20140. Medline:20461783

Widespread pain

7

Rheumatologic Manifestations of Medical Disease

DR. MICHAEL G. BLACKMORE
UNIVERSITY OF TORONTO

KEY CONCEPTS

1. Rheumatologic complaints secondary to underlying chronic medical disorders can produce significant morbidity in patients.
2. Musculoskeletal complaints may be the initial presentation of a wide variety of diseases.
3. Rheumatologic problems can be due to the disease process itself or can be secondary to metabolic derangement associated with the disease. There may be other unexplained associations.

Endocrine Disorders

DIABETES MELLITUS

Many musculoskeletal manifestations of diabetes are thought to be due to microvascular abnormalities, with damage to blood vessels and nerves, glycosylation of collagen, and accumulation of abnormal collagen in skin and periarticular structures.

The following section shows 1 scheme for organizing the musculoskeletal manifestations of diabetes.[1]

Conditions unique to diabetes mellitus

Diabetic muscle infarction: This is rare and presents as a localized, exquisitely painful swelling with limited range of motion of the lower extremity. It is self-limited.

Diabetic amyotrophy: This is a lumbosacral plexopathy with some involvement of lumbosacral nerve roots and peripheral nerves. It characteristically produces acute, asymmetrical pain, followed by weakness involving the proximal leg with associated weight loss and autonomic dysfunction. It is likely due to ischemic neuropathy secondary to microvascular disease.

Mononeuritis multiplex: This can mimic vasculitis (and should be excluded before attributing mononeuritis multiplex to an inflammatory vasculitis).

Diabetic sclerodactyly: This involves thickening and waxiness of the skin that is seen mainly on fingers. It can look like scleroderma, but there is no Raynaud phenomena, ulcers, etc. It may be associated with cheiroarthropathy (see below).

Conditions occurring more frequently in diabetes mellitus

Trigger fingers, flexor tenosynovitis, and stenosing tenosynovitis: These are characterized by palpable nodule formation and thickening of the flexor tendon or sheath. Triggering or locking phenomena are associated with this.

Dupuytren contracture

Diabetic cheiroarthropathy (syndrome of limited joint mobility): This presents with insidious onset of contractures and stiffening of the hands.

The underlying deposition of abnormal collagen in connective tissue around the joints may also lead to skin changes that look like scleroderma (see diabetic sclerodactyly, above). Affected individuals will not be able to flatten the palm and/or fingers against the surface of a table or flatten the hands together as in prayer ("prayer sign").

Adhesive capsulitis or frozen shoulder: This presents with insidious onset of pain (especially at nighttime, with difficulty lying on the affected side) and marked impairment of range of motion of the shoulder. On examination, reduction in active and passive abduction and external rotation is characteristic. It requires physiotherapy and nonsteroidal anti-inflammatory drugs (NSAIDs) (often problematic in patients with diabetes mellitus) or intra-articular glucocorticoid injection.

Carpal tunnel syndrome

Septic arthritis: Patients with diabetes have an increased risk of this condition.

Diabetic arthropathy secondary to neuropathy: This is also known as Charcot joint and is a rare complication.

Conditions sharing risk factors of diabetes mellitus and metabolic syndrome

Gout

Osteoarthritis

Diffuse idiopathic skeletal hyperostosis (DISH): This is characterized by the formation of bridging enthesophytes in the spine, as well as enthesophytes and osteophytes in peripheral joints. Affected joints "stiffen up" with reduced range of motion.

THYROID DISEASE

Musculoskeletal problems are common in thyroid disease, and may be the first—and sometimes only—clinical sign of thyroid disease. Thus, it is important to screen for thyroid dysfunction among people with musculoskeletal presentations, as thyroid diseases are easy to diagnose and generally easily treated. The musculoskeletal manifestations tend to resolve when a euthyroid state is reached.

Hypothyroidism

Symmetrical arthropathy of hands and/or knees: This tends to be noninflammatory. It may be related to calcium pyrophosphate dihydrate (CPPD) deposition, but can look like rheumatoid arthritis (RA).

Asymptomatic chondrocalcinosis and clinical pseudogout

Proximal myopathy (see chapter 3): This may be associated with elevated CK.

Carpal tunnel syndrome: This can be bilateral, which may be a clue to the underlying disorder.

Hyperthyroidism

Proximal myopathy: This can be severe. CK may not be elevated.

Adhesive capsulitis of the shoulders: This is typically bilateral.

Osteoporosis

Pretibial myxedema: This presents as skin induration over the pretibial area.

PARATHYROID DISEASE

Hyperparathyroidism

Osteoporosis

Chondrocalcinosis and pseudogout

Vague myalgias and malaise: Myopathy is possible.

Bone disease with cysts, erosions, and deformities

Tendon ruptures

Hypoparathyroidism

- This may lead to ossification of paraspinal ligaments. It can produce a syndrome that looks like ankylosing spondylitis (but there is no sacroiliitis and it does not respond to NSAIDs).

- It can also look similar to DISH with paravertebral ossification. The mechanism of these skeletal abnormalities is not well defined.

- A myopathy has also been described.

CUSHING SYNDROME AND EXOGENOUS CUSHING SYNDROME

Osteoporosis

Avascular necrosis

Proximal myopathy

Chronic Kidney Disease

Chronic musculoskeletal pain is common in patients with chronic kidney disease, both early and late stage.

Renal osteodystrophy

- This is part of the larger category of chronic kidney disease mineral-and bone-related disorders (CKD-MBD).

- The driving factor is phosphate retention, which leads to increased calcium binding, causing serum hypocalcemia.

- Decreased activation of vitamin D in the kidney also contributes to hypocalcemia (reduced gastrointestinal absorption).

- Compensatory hyperparathyroidism ensues, which results in increased bone turnover with increased osteoclastic activity and bone resorption at subperiosteal, subchondral, and subligamentous or subtendinous sites. This may also contribute to the destructive changes seen in amyloid arthropathy (see below). Subperiosteal resorption can be seen early on X-ray and is pathognomonic of hyperparathyroidism. It may become extensive and involve SI joints, intervertebral discs, and other areas, mimicking ankylosing spondylitis.

- Other features are bone mineralization abnormalities (osteomalacia) and adynamic bone disease and osteopenia.

Extraskeletal calcification

- This complication is the result of the raised calcium-phosphorus product together with the effects of exogenous calcium and vitamin D intake in the presence of adynamic bone disease.

- It may present with cartilaginous deposits presenting with chondrocalcinosis in knee, wrist, hip, and shoulders.

- Calcification may occur in periarticular areas as well, producing radiographic cloud-like densities around hip, shoulder, elbow, knee, small hand and foot joints, bursae, tendons, and ligaments.

Amyloid arthropathy

- Increased synthesis and retention of β_2-microglobulin in patients on hemodialysis produces a secondary form of amyloidosis.

- Amyloid arthropathy is characterized by erosive osteoarthropathies, destructive spondyloarthropathy, and carpal tunnel syndrome.

- Secondary hyperparathyroidism, CPPD crystal deposition, and metabolic bone disease probably contribute to the development of these problems.

- In the small joints, amyloid arthropathy can look like RA with erosive lesions appearing on X-ray (but not periarticular osteopenia as would be seen in RA).

Spontaneous tendon rupture

- This problem can be seen in patients on long-term hemodialysis and renal transplantation.
- It may be due to changes in tendon strength in the setting of chronic uremia, associated hyperparathyroidism affecting the entheses, the presence of amyloidosis, glucocorticoid therapy, and the use of fluoroquinolone antibiotics.
- Classic locations include the Achilles, quadriceps, and rotator cuff tendons.

Osteonecrosis
Infection

- There is increased risk of septic arthritis and osteomyelitis due to chronic disease with relative immunosuppression, and with a portal of entry via dialysis in those receiving renal replacement therapy.

Gout

- Renal insufficiency leads to reduced excretion of urate and hyperuricemia. Recurrent gouty attacks are common in patients with chronic kidney disease. Dialysis usually resolves this problem.
- Renal transplantation may be associated with hyperuricemia secondary to use of calcineurin inhibitors (cyclosporine, tacrolimus) as immunomodulators.

Nephrogenic systemic fibrosis

- This is a gadolinium-induced fibrotic process mainly affecting skin and internal organs in patients with impaired renal function who are exposed to gadolinium while undergoing an MRI scan.

- Skin changes include thickening and woody induration of the skin with yellowish or brownish discolouration associated with burning and pruritus.
- The conditions does **not** present with Raynaud phenomenon, nail fold capillary changes, telangiectasia, etc., as would be seen with scleroderma.

HIV/AIDS

There has been a decline in the prevalence of HIV/AIDS and a decline in AIDS-associated deaths. However, the World Health Organization estimates that roughly 35 million people are living with HIV. Globally, there are still approximately 2 million new infections per year.

While mortality has decreased in the era of highly active antiretroviral therapy (HAART), AIDS morbidity has increased because individuals are now living with chronic disease and the effects of treatment. Rheumatic conditions can be a significant cause of morbidity in people living with HIV/AIDS. This is thought to be the result of depletion of CD4+ T cells, inversion of the CD4+/CD8+ T-lymphocyte ratio, and development of antibodies that favour immune complex formation (through constant exposure to HIV antigens). Treatment with HAART can result in a paradoxical immune reconstitution inflammatory syndrome (IRIS) that may be associated with a new or reactivated autoimmune or rheumatologic disease (which was quiescent during the period of CD4 T-cell depletion).

The management of rheumatic diseases in the HIV-infected individual is similar to that of noninfected individuals. Greater caution should be used with immunosuppressive medications and individuals should be closely monitored for opportunistic infections. Particular care must be used if CD4 values are lower than 200 cells/μL.

HIV arthralgia and arthritis

- This affects approximately 5% of HIV-infected people.
- Its duration is less than 6 weeks.
- It can be oligoarticular or polyarticular.
- Synovial fluid cultures are negative.
- Results for antinuclear antibody and rheumatoid factor are negative.
- A chronic, erosive process with radiographic change can be seen (less common).
- Note that joint pain may be secondary to **avascular necrosis**.
  - Both HIV itself (especially with very low CD4 cell counts) and HAART are risk factors.
  - Patients receiving glucocorticoids for management of rheumatic condition may be at higher risk.
- Chronic widespread pain due to fibromyalgia (see chapter 6) has also been described.

Spondylarthritis

- Increase in undifferentiated spondylarthritis is associated with the AIDS epidemic of the 1980s.
- The presentation tends to be predominantly arthritis (lower extremity) and enthesitis with less spondylitis.
- Psoriasis and psoriatic arthritis can be severe, but improve with HAART.

- Treatment is similar to that for noninfected individuals. Tumour necrosis factor inhibitors have been used successfully.

Rheumatoid arthritis

- This tends to remit in HIV-infected patients because of decreased CD4 T cells.
- New-onset RA is rare in the context of HIV infection.
- With HAART, immune reconstitution phenomenon may worsen RA that was quiescent during the low CD4 state, or allow new onset of disease.

Serological abnormalities

- Patients with HIV have multiple serological abnormalities: hypergammaglobulinemia, positive rheumatoid factor, antineutrophil cytoplasmic antibodies, antinuclear antibodies, anticardiolipin antibodies.
- This should be considered in patients being worked up for possible connective tissue disease (see chapter 5b).
- These antibodies are rarely of clinical significance.

Systemic lupus erythematosus

- This is similar to the situation with RA.
- It is generally quiescent in patients with HIV infection but may become activated during immune reconstitution.

Diffuse infiltrative lymphocytosis syndrome (DILS) (Sjögren-like syndrome)

- This affects 3% to 4% of HIV-infected people, but has decreased with HAART.
- It presents with bilateral enlargement of parotid, submandibular, or lacrimal glands.

Endo/Renal/HIV

- It is typically present with sicca symptoms (dry mouth, dry eyes), but has negative Ro/La antibody results (and pathological features distinct from Sjögren syndrome).
- Extraglandular involvement may include pneumonitis, cranial nerve VII palsy, peripheral neuropathy, polymyositis (PM), renal tubular acidosis, hepatitis, and lymphoma.
- In an HIV-infected patient with parotid enlargement, also consider malignancy and granulomatous disease.

Vasculitis

- The full range of vasculitic diseases is seen in HIV-infected individuals, with presentations similar to those in noninfected individuals.
- Polyarteritis nodosa (PAN) has been reported, as well as antineutrophil cytoplasmic antibody–associated small vessel vasculitis, Henoch-Schönlein purpura, and Behçet disease (see chapter 5a).
- Drug-induced cutaneous vasculitis has been reported.
- Traditional therapy for vasculitis (prednisone or cyclophosphamide) seems to be successful.

Myopathy

- Polymyositis (PM) in this context is similar to idiopathic PM (see chapter 3).
  - Prevalence is reported as high as 0.25%.
  - Anti-Jo-1 and Mi-2 antibodies are absent. The condition may have normal electromyography and biopsy results; thus, clinical evaluation is important (maintain index of suspicion).
  - It responds well to standard therapy for PM, as in non-HIV patients.

- Other myopathies include DILS, inclusion-body myositis, and others.
- In the differential diagnosis for myopathy in HIV-infected patients, also consider infection (pyomyositis) or rhabdomyolysis associated with HAART.

Rheumatologic manifestations of HIV therapy

- The integrase inhibitor, raltegravir, can be associated with severe rhabdomyolysis and acute renal failure, as can other protease inhibitors. Be watchful in patients also receiving statins.
- Indinavir has been associated with adhesive capsulitis, Dupuytren contracture, tenosynovitis, and temporomandibular malfunction.
- Immune reconstitution inflammation syndrome (IRIS), associated with successful HAART can result in the appearance of autoimmune diseases de novo, or the reactivation of a disease that was previously quiescent during the period of immunosuppression.
- IRIS occurs approximately 9 months from initiation of HAART.

Musculoskeletal infections

- *Staphylococcus aureus* is still the most common pathogen in acute musculoskeletal infection (septic arthritis, osteomyelitis, pyomyositis).
- Atypical mycobacterial bone and joint infections are well described in patients with advanced immunosuppression in the setting of HIV infection and may present with a more indolent picture.

Endo/Renal/HIV

Reference

1. Bañón S, Isenberg DA. Rheumatological manifestations occurring in patients with diabetes mellitus. *Scand J Rheumatol.* 2013;42(1):1–10. http://dx.doi.org/10.3109/03009742.2012.713983. Medline:23130978

Further Reading

Bardin T. Musculoskeletal manifestations of chronic renal failure. *Curr Opin Rheumatol*. 2003;15(1):48–54. http://dx.doi.org/10.1097/00002281-200301000-00009. Medline:12496510

Chakravarty SD, Markenson JA. Rheumatic manifestations of endocrine disease. *Curr Opin Rheumatol*. 2013;25(1):37–43. http://dx.doi.org/10.1097/BOR.0b013e32835b4f3f. Medline:23159916

Lim CY, Ong KO. Various musculoskeletal manifestations of chronic renal insufficiency. *Clin Radiol*. 2013;68(7):e397–411. http://dx.doi.org/10.1016/j.crad.2013.01.025. Medline:23522485

Maganti RM, Reveille JD, Williams FM. Therapy insight: the changing spectrum of rheumatic disease in HIV infection. *Nat Clin Pract Rheumatol*. 2008;4(8):428–38. http://dx.doi.org/10.1038/ncprheum0836. Medline:18577999

Nguyen BY, Reveille JD. Rheumatic manifestations associated with HIV in the highly active antiretroviral therapy era. *Curr Opin Rheumatol*. 2009;21(4):404–10. http://dx.doi.org/10.1097/BOR.0b013e32832c9d04. Medline:19444116

8

Back Pain

DR. LORI ALBERT
UNIVERSITY OF TORONTO

KEY CONCEPTS

1. Low back pain is common and can be disabling.
2. Back pain is typically seen in active and otherwise healthy people.
3. Most back pain in general practice is mechanical, in which the pain arises from a structural element or elements within the spine. It is usually not possible to determine the precise source of pain.
4. History is important to establish the pattern of pain: recognizing distinct patterns of reliable historical and clinical features allows back pain to be categorized and managed.
5. History is also critical to address "red flags" by probing for significant neurologic compromise or serious underlying disease, particularly when the patient's symptoms do not fit a mechanical pattern.
6. Less than 5% of back pain is secondary to seronegative inflammatory spondylarthritis (SpA), but this is an important cause of pain in younger individuals. Back pain is **not** a feature of rheumatoid arthritis or other seropositive arthritis.
7. In the absence of red flags, conservative management of back pain is successful in most cases.

History

PATIENT DEMOGRAPHICS

- Low back pain is a common symptom that reflects a heterogeneous clinical entity. Among adults, 60% to 80% will suffer from at least 1 episode of back pain during their lifetime.

- Risk factors include older age; heavy labour, especially jobs requiring lifting in an awkward position; lower education and income; smoking; and obesity.

- Prior episodes of back pain are strong predictors of recurrence.

- Back pain in patients older than 50 (for the first episode) or younger than 20 should raise the index of suspicion for a more serious pathological condition.

KEY QUESTIONS

Global approach

One approach to back pain history is to determine which of the "4 patterns" of back pain best fit the patient's symptoms. It is accepted that this is a reliable way to exclude serious conditions.[1,2] This determination will also help guide the approach to therapy. Key questions include those required to rule out a significant medical cause of back pain or neurologic compromise.

The pathophysiology of most nonspecific (mechanical) back pain is not well understood (but this lack of understanding does not undermine the management approach). Therefore, in evaluating patients presenting with low back pain, focus on determining whether the pattern of pain fits into one of the 4 recognized patterns (Table 8.1).

TABLE 8.1. Mechanical patterns of back pain

Back-dominant pain Pain is felt most intensely in or over the back, buttock, coccyx, greater trochanter, groin.	Pattern 1: Discogenic	Pattern 2: Posterior elements
History	Pain is constant or intermittent. It is worse with flexion.	Pain is intermittent. It is increased with back extension, never with flexion.
Physical	Pain is increased with back flexion. Neurologic examination is normal.	Pain is increased with back extension. Neurologic examination is normal.
Leg-dominant pain Pain is felt around or below the gluteal fold and can extend to the thigh, calf, ankle, foot	Pattern 3: Sciatica	Pattern 4: Neurogenic claudication
History	Pain is constant (leg pain). Leg pain location on examination matches history.	Pain is intermittent. It is increased with activity in extension, relieved with flexion
Physical	There are positive neurologic findings ordinarily (nerve root irritation test, conduction loss).	Nerve root irritation tests are negative; nerve conduction loss may be found.

Adapted with permission from Dr. H. Hall.

Back pain

Key questions to determine whether low back pain fits into a recognized mechanical pattern

1. Where is your pain the worst? Establish whether is it back-dominant or leg-dominant pain.

2. Is the pain intermittent or constant?

3. Is the pain worse with bending forward (flexion)?

4. Since the start of your pain, has there been any change in bowel or bladder function? Loss of bowel or bladder function is a red flag indicating a more serious condition.

5. What can't you do now that you could do before your pain and why? Persistent significant functional limitation could indicate a more serious cause for pain.

6. What are the relieving movements or positions?

7. Have you had this type of pain before? Recurrent episodes are more consistent with a mechanical pattern.

8. Have you had treatment in the past and was it effective?

If the patient's symptoms do not fit into one of the 4 patterns, then other systemic, serious causes for back pain should be sought.

Nonmechanical back pain
Nonmechanical spine disease includes the following:

- malignancy (e.g., multiple myeloma, metastatic carcinoma, other tumours)
- infection (e.g., osteomyelitis, septic discitis, epidural abscess, paraspinal abscess)
- hemorrhage (e.g., epidural hematoma)
- compression fracture
- inflammatory arthritis of the spine (e.g., ankylosing spondylitis and other forms of SpA)

Back pain can also be **referred from viscera** (e.g., nephrolithiasis, dissecting aneurysm, pelvic disease).

Key questions to identify nonmechanical causes of back pain: red flags
1. Is there pain that is constant and/or is there night or recumbency pain? These symptoms

suggest tumour, inflammation from infection, or ankylosing spondylitis (AS).

2. Has there been recent-onset bladder dysfunction such as urinary retention, increased frequency, overflow incontinence, bowel incontinence, or saddle anesthesia? These symptoms suggest cauda equina syndrome.

3. Are there constitutional symptoms such as fever, chills, or unexplained weight loss? These symptoms suggest tumour, infection, or possibly inflammatory disease.

4. Has there been any recent infection (especially urinary tract infection in elderly patients), IV drug abuse, immune suppression (steroids, transplant, or HIV), or risk factors for tuberculosis?

5. Is there a history of malignancy?

6. Is there a history of trauma? This can be relatively minor, or it can even be a history of strenuous lifting in a potentially osteoporotic individual (see chapter 9).

7. Is there any use of anticoagulants? Consider epidural bleed.

Key questions to identify inflammatory SpA

Several sets of criteria exist that are designed to maximize sensitivity and specificity for the diagnosis of inflammatory back pain. The criteria endorsed by the Assessment of Spondylarthritis International Society (ASAS) include the following 5 findings:

- age of onset younger than 45 years
- insidious onset of symptoms
- improvement with exercise
- no improvement with rest
- pain at night (with improvement upon getting up)

Back pain

A result of at least 4 positive answers has a sensitivity of 79.6% and a specificity of 72.4% (but the predictive value may be low because of the relative rarity of disease).

Additional history if considering spondylitis

- Inquire about the following:
  - pain with duration longer than 3 months
  - morning stiffness
  - midthoracic pain
  - peripheral arthritis and enthesitis
  - alternating buttock pain (reflecting sacroiliitis)
  - improvement of pain with anti-inflammatory drug (NSAID) therapy
  - extra-articular manifestations (e.g., psoriasis, uveitis, and inflammatory bowel disease)

- Also inquire about a family history of AS, psoriasis, and inflammatory bowel disease, as all can be relevant to a presenting complaint suggesting inflammatory back disease.

Physical Examination

General appearance: Assess the patient's overall presentation (sick or well), degree of pain, exaggerated pain behaviour, antalgic gait.

Vital signs: If the patient has a fever or tachycardia, consider infection or serious medical cause.

Head and neck: Check for ocular inflammation, oral ulcers, psoriasis in scalp (all are seen with SpA).

Chest: Check for chest wall tenderness, sternomanubrial tenderness, reduction in chest wall expansion (suggesting SpA).

Cardiovascular exam: Asymmetrical pulses may indicate aortic dissection or vascular claudication as a cause of leg pain.

Abdomen: Tenderness or enlargement of viscera may be a cause of pain. Enlarged aneurysm may be a cause.

Back exam: See the section that follows.

PROCEDURES FOR BACK EXAMINATION

This involves 4 separate procedures:

- regional back examination
- neurologic screening
- tests for sciatic nerve tension and irritation
- examination for SpA (when suggested by history)

Regional back examination

- Look for limping, or coordination suggesting neurologic impairment.
- Vertebral point tenderness to palpation may suggest spinal fracture, infection, or tumour with the associated clinical picture. Palpation is best done with the patient in the prone position with a pillow under the abdomen to relax paraspinal muscles and reduce the lumbar lordosis.
- Pain with direct pressure over SI joints may support a history suggestive of sacroiliitis.
- Check range of motion (flexion, extension, lateral flexion).
- Guarding that occurs in all planes of movement suggests an infection, tumour, or fracture (but this is not reliable without a very strong supporting clinical picture). Global reduction in range of motion may also be seen with inflammatory disease, usually after a more prolonged history of back pain.

Neurologic examination

- Focus on a few tests to look for nerve root impairment (see Table 8.2).

TABLE 8.2. Simplified neurologic examination for assessing patients with back pain

	Nerve root being tested		
	L4	**L5**	**S1**
Location of pain	Anterolateral thigh and shin	Buttock, lateral thigh and leg, dorsum foot	Buttock, back of thigh and leg, lateral foot
Sensory screening	Reduced pinprick sensation on medial aspect of foot	Reduced pinprick sensation on dorsal foot	Reduced pinprick sensation on lateral aspect of foot
Motor weakness testing	Extension of quadriceps: test with patient seated; extend knee against resistance	Dorsiflexion of great toe and foot: test with patient seated, foot on floor; elevate great toe against resistance; elevate forefoot against resistance	Plantar flexion of great toe and foot: test with patient seated, foot on floor
		Hip abduction (Trendelenburg test): while standing, patient raises 1 leg and then the other; test the hip abductors of the leg on which the patient is standing	Plantar flexion: patent raises toes on both feet and then on the affected side
			Gluteus maximus: test with patient prone; palpate buttocks as patient tenses and relaxes
Motor weakness screening manoeuvre	Squat and rise	Heel walking (L4): walk 5 steps	Toe walking: walk 5 steps
Reflexes	Knee jerk diminished (test with patient seated, lower leg hanging free)	None reliable (sometimes medial hamstring reflex if absent on affected side)	Ankle jerk diminished (may need to test with patient kneeling)

Pearl: More than 90% of clinically significant lower extremity radiculopathies involve the L5 or S1 nerve root at the L4–L5 or L5–S1 disc levels, respectively.

- Look for evidence of muscle atrophy by comparing circumferential measurements of the calf and thigh bilaterally. Asymmetry will be seen in neurologic impairment or if there is a preexisting joint problem (e.g., hamstring and anterior compartment wasting for long-standing S1 root injuries).

- Complete the 2 essential components of a neurologic examination to detect upper motor and low sacral root involvement:
  - **Look for up-going toes (positive Babinski sign) or clonus**, which may indicate upper motor-neuron abnormalities (such as myelopathy or demyelinating disease) and exclude a simple mechanical low back diagnosis.
  - **Look for saddle anesthesia** involving the buttocks, posterior-superior thighs, and perineal region to test lower sacral roots. You can test in the midline between the upper buttocks. Also assess for reduced anal sphincter tone, if indicated.

Tests for sciatic nerve tension and irritation

Straight leg raising (SLR): supine

- Cup the patient's heel in 1 hand and, keeping the knee fully extended with the other hand, slowly raise the straight leg from the examining table until pain occurs.
- Tension is transmitted to the nerve roots once the leg is raised beyond 30°, but after 70°, further movement of the nerve is negligible, and movement of the pelvis occurs because of stretch of the hamstrings.
- A positive test result reproduces sciatica symptoms between 30° and 60° of leg elevation.
- You can confirm a positive result with dorsiflexion of the foot. This should aggravate symptoms, even if the elevation of the foot is reduced by 10° to 15°.

Back pain

- **Note that reproducing pain in the back with SLR is not a positive test.**
- The final phase of testing involves dorsiflexion of the foot after reducing elevation of the foot by a further 10° to 15°. This should not aggravate symptoms, as tension has been reduced on the nerve. Reproduction of back pain is not relevant.
- A crossed SLR occurs when SLR is performed on the unaffected leg and is found to elicit pain in the symptomatic leg. This has increased specificity for a herniated disc.

Straight leg raising (SLR): sitting
- With the patient sitting on a table, and both hips and knees flexed at 90°, slowly extend the knee. This manoeuvre stretches nerve roots, and the patient with significant nerve root irritation will complain or lean backward to reduce tension on the nerve.
- Do a **femoral stretch test** when suggested by history. The patient is prone with the knee extended. The examiner passively lifts the leg. Reproduction or exacerbation of anterior thigh (L2–L3) or medial leg (L4) pain is a positive test and indicates nerve root irritation at the levels indicated. Production of back pain is common but not relevant.

Back examination for inflammatory SpA
The physical examination of the back is of limited discriminant value in the initial assessment of a patient with inflammatory back pain. However, range of motion of the lumbar spine may be reduced with AS and related conditions.

Schober test
- Place a mark with a pen at the lumbosacral junction (just above the dimples of Venus) and a mark 10 cm above.

- With forward flexion, the distance between the marks should increase to 15 cm.

Lateral spinal flexion

- The patient stands with their back against a wall, hands down and extended, resting against the lateral thighs. On each thigh in turn, make a mark at the tip of the third finger.
- The patient bends laterally as far as possible, keeping their back against the wall. Make a mark at the new location of the tip of the third finger.
- A distance between the 2 marks of less than 10 cm is clearly abnormal (this test can also be done by measuring the distance from the tip of the third finger to the floor in the neutral and then the side-bending position).

Chest expansion

- The patient puts their hands on their head. Place a tape measure tightly around the patient's chest at the level of the xiphisternum.
- Ask the patient to inhale deeply, and then exhale fully.
- Tighten the tape measure and ask the patient to inhale fully once more.
- Chest circumference from end-expiration to end-inspiration should be 5 to 6 cm.
- A measurement less than 3 cm is clearly abnormal.

Range of motion of cervical spine

- Position the patient prone or seated. Stand behind the patient to visualize the vertex of the patient's head.
- The patient rotates their head from neutral position to full rotation, first on 1 side and then the other.

- Using the top of the nose as an indicator, estimate the degrees of movement from the neutral position.
- Precise measurement can be done by using a goniometer with 1 arm of the measuring device stabilized against your body and the fulcrum aligned with the vertex of the patient's skull. The free arm rotates to follow the patient's rotation and the degrees of movement can be measured.

Occiput-to-wall and tragus-to-wall distance
- Position the patient with their heels and back resting against a wall. The patient holds their chin at its usual carrying level.
- The patient makes maximal effort to touch their head against the wall without tilting the chin up.
- Measure the distance from the most prominent part of the occiput or the tip of the tragus to the wall.
- The occiput-to-wall distance is normally 0 cm; the tragus-to-wall distance is normally 10 cm.

Stress manoeuvres for SI joint inflammation
- These are poorly reproducible and inaccurate in distinguishing inflammatory from mechanical spine problems:
  - **FABER (flexion, abduction, and external rotation with distracting force):** The patient is supine, and places the heel of 1 foot against opposite knee. The examiner presses against the knee and opposite anterior superior iliac spine of pelvis. Pain elicited in the SI joint ipsilateral to the flexed knee is considered a positive result.
  - **Gaenslen (hyperextension of hip/leg):** The patient is supine, lying at the edge of a bed. The leg is gently lowered off the bed into hyperextension,

while the pelvis is stabilized by the patient holding their contralateral knee flexed against chest. Pain in the SI joint of the hyperextended leg is considered a positive result.

- **Lateral compression:** The patient is lying on their side. The examiner places their weight, through extended arms, on the lateral pelvis of the patient. Pain in the inferior SI joint (side on the table) is considered a positive result.

- Always check for **enthesitis** by palpating the Achilles tendon insertion at the calcaneus, palpating the plantar fascia insertion at the calcaneus, and palpating for tenderness at the pelvic brim. Other sites include the quadriceps insertion into the patella, the patellar ligament insertion into the tibial tuberosity, the medial and lateral epicondyles, the greater trochanter of the femur, and the supraspinatus tendon insertion into the greater tuberosity of the humerus.

Key Laboratory Testing

Consider the following tests for patients in whom mechanical back pain is less likely (i.e., first onset of back pain occurs before age 50, or pain has concerning features on history or physical examination).

CBC

ESR: Look for very high ESR, suggesting malignancy or inflammation from infection or AS.

Alkaline phosphatase, calcium

Serum protein electrophoresis

Urine/blood cultures: Pursue these as indicated.

HLA-B27 testing:

- This is rarely helpful as a diagnostic tool in the setting of chronic back pain.

- Ordering HLA-B27 should be restricted to those cases where the pretest probability that the patient has SpA is intermediate on the basis of a history compatible with inflammatory back pain, or in cases where there are other features of SpA (e.g., enthesitis, uveitis, asymmetrical peripheral arthritis, positive family history).

- Patients who have clearly abnormal SI joints on imaging (see "Imaging" below), along with a compatible history, do not necessarily need to have HLA-B27 testing, as the diagnosis of seronegative SpA can be confirmed without it.

- On the other hand, some patients never develop radiographic sacroiliitis, or develop changes only over many years. In a patient with at least 2 SpA features, HLA-B27 can be checked, as this could support the clinical diagnosis of SpA (see "Differential Diagnosis" below).

Imaging

Imaging, in a nontrauma setting, carries a lack of specificity.

- Imaging abnormalities frequently do not correlate with specific symptoms, pain severity, or degree of disability.

- Imaging does not improve patient outcomes for those with a mechanical pattern of pain.

- Imaging does not typically permit pinpointing of the pain generator in a particular individual, but spinal imaging does increase costs.

When the history raises concerns for more serious pathology, judicious use of imaging will assist in the diagnosis of spinal tumours, infections, and fractures. The role of imaging when there is suspicion for SpA is important.

Plain X-rays:

- Pelvic radiographs can confirm the diagnosis of SpA when they demonstrate definitive sacroiliitis in the patient with back pain of more than 3 months duration plus at least 1 other feature of SpA (peripheral arthritis, enthesitis, uveitis, positive family history, etc.).

  - Standard anteroposterior radiographs may not allow for good visualization of the SI joint because of its oblique orientation.
  - Request an oblique view, which is a 30° cephalad angled view.
  - Pelvic X-rays also allow visualization of the hip joints, which are frequently affected in SpA (especially AS).
  - Structural changes of sacroiliitis can take many years to develop, and this can contribute to the delay in diagnosis of AS. In such settings, MRI may be useful in detecting "nonradiographic" SpA (see "Differential Diagnosis" below).

- Radiographic evaluation of the spine in established SpA may reveal changes related to ossification of the spinal ligaments that bridge the intervertebral discs, which leads to characteristic vertically oriented bony outgrowths called syndesmophytes. In AS, you may also see "squaring" of the vertebral bodies induced by osteitis and subsequent erosions of the anterior, superior, and inferior surfaces of the vertebrae, followed by reparative new bone formation.

- Degenerative changes in the spine seen on plain X-ray are extremely common and rarely advance the diagnosis of back pain. These changes include disc space narrowing, vertebral "lipping," osteophytes (horizontally oriented compared with the vertically oriented syndesmophytes), end-plate sclerosis and cysts, and mild degrees of anterolisthesis.

CT scan: This may demonstrate more convincing changes of sacroiliitis when pelvic X-rays are equivocal, but increased radiation exposure limits its use in routine clinical practice. CT scans may better define bony lesions than plain X-rays or MRI.

MRI:

- MRI better defines soft tissue in setting of suspected disc herniation, as well as paraspinal disease. This is the preferred test if cauda equina syndrome or myelopathy is suspected.

- MRI is the only imaging modality that can provide an early diagnosis of sacroiliitis, before radiographic changes are evident.

  - The characteristic change is bone marrow edema, which appears hypointense (**dark**) on T1-weighted images and hyperintense (**bright**) on fluid-sensitive short tau inversion recovery (STIR) images or on T2-weighted images with fat signal suppression. **Note:** These images should be specifically requested.
  - Gadolinium contrast may aid in identifying inflammatory lesions; on fat-suppressed T1-weighted images, contrast enhancement of the subchondral bone may be seen.
  - Similar changes may be seen elsewhere in the spine when active spondylitis is present.

- Note that some patients may never develop radiographic sacroiliitis, but can be diagnosed with SpA on the basis of clinical criteria (see the section that follows: "Differential Diagnosis").

RADIOGRAPHIC SACROILIITIS

Grade 0 = normal

Grade 1 = suspicious changes

Grade 2 = minimal abnormality (small localized areas with erosion or sclerosis, without alteration in the joint width)

Grade 3 = unequivocal abnormality (moderate or advanced sacroiliitis with erosions, evidence of sclerosis, widening, narrowing, or partial ankylosis)

Grade 4 = severe abnormality (total ankylosis)

Differential Diagnosis

Consider the possibility of referred or visceral causes of back pain in the following:

- disease of visceral organs (pancreatitis, cholecystitis, etc.)
- dissecting aneurysm
- myocardial infarction

In acute back or leg-dominant pain, consider the possibility of herpes zoster and examine the patient for characteristic skin lesions.

NOTE ON DIAGNOSIS OF SPA

In 2009, the ASAS classification criteria for axial SpA were published. Entry into this algorithm requires patients to have back pain of more than 3 months duration with onset before age 45. These patients can be classified as having axial SpA based on the following:

- **Imaging criteria:** sacroiliitis present on MRI *or* on X-ray *and* at least 1 SpA feature
- **Clinical criteria:** HLA-B27 positivity *and* at least 2 SpA features[3]

SPA FEATURES
Inflammatory back pain
Arthritis
Enthesitis (heel)
Uveitis
Dactylitis
Psoriasis
Crohn disease/colitis
Good response to NSAIDs
Family history for SpA
HLA-B27
Elevated CRP

Treatment Options

Back surgery is warranted in fewer than 5% of people with back pain.

MECHANICAL BACK PAIN

- A conservative approach is warranted, with a focus on mechanical measures, self-care modalities (heat, ice, etc.) and first-line analgesics (acetaminophen, NSAIDs) to permit moderate exercise. There is some evidence for the role of spinal manipulation in management of acute low back pain for patients who do not improve with self-care options.

- Education enables patients to understand the expected course of this condition. Mechanical back pain is common, not dangerous, and largely self-limited, but may recur.

  - Patients can also learn techniques to prevent and manage flares.
  - A similar approach may be used for chronic mechanical back pain, with a focus on improving function and controlling symptoms (though the patient may not be "cured").
  - There should also be a focus on self-reliance, rather than supervised care, in managing

symptoms. Patients should avoid aggravating activities, and develop a regular exercise routine.

- Other modalities such as massage, acupuncture, yoga, and relaxation therapy have some support in the literature.
- Guidelines exist in the literature for management of both acute and chronic low back pain.

- In the acute/subacute setting, reevaluation is warranted after 4 to 8 weeks of conservative therapy. The patient who fails to respond may need to be reassessed for a more serious underlying cause of pain.

BACK PAIN WITH NERVE ROOT OR CORD INVOLVEMENT

- For patients with acute leg-dominant pain, consistent with radiculopathy, a conservative approach is also prudent, given that 80% of cases resolve spontaneously.

  - Stronger analgesics may be required (i.e., opioid analgesics) or drugs used for neuropathic pain, such as antidepressants or antiseizure medications.
  - Patients may be able to identify rest positions where pain is relieved (such as lying on the floor with legs resting on a chair seat).
  - Imaging by MRI is recommended only if the patient is under serious consideration for an intervention such as surgery or epidural steroid injection, or in the presence of more severe or progressive neurologic deficits.

- Cauda equina syndrome is an indication for urgent intervention: a surgical consultation is required if due to a massive posterior disc herniation or bleed; a radiation therapy consultation is needed in the setting of a malignant lesion.

- Management of neurogenic claudication is focused on maintaining or restoring function due to the underlying spinal stenosis, rather than focusing on the leg pain, which is generally intermittent. This will usually involve some form of physiotherapy and other measures such as maintenance of a healthy weight, modifications to provocative activities, etc.

BACK PAIN SECONDARY TO OTHER MEDICAL CAUSES

- Treatment of infection or a malignant lesion depends on the nature of the process and should be undertaken with the input of appropriate consultants.

- Treatment of osteoporotic fractures is usually conservative, but should be an indication for medical management of osteoporosis if not already in place (see chapter 9).

SPONDYLARTHRITIS

- Management of SpA can be complex and should be undertaken with the input of a rheumatology consultant.

- Nonpharmacologic interventions include education, regular exercise, and physiotherapy to maintain posture and function.

- The primary pharmacologic option is NSAIDs, used continuously for persistent active and symptomatic disease.

- Patients who do not respond adequately to a trial of least 2 NSAIDs are candidates for "biologic" therapy with tumour necrosis factor (TNF) inhibitors.

- There is no evidence to support the use of systemic glucocorticoids or nonbiologic disease-modifying antirheumatic drugs (DMARDs such as methotrexate and sulfasalazine) in the axial component of AS. TNF inhibitors are the only class of biologics currently approved for AS. If the back pain is attributable to AS, TNF inhibitors will be effective in controlling symptoms in more than 70% of treated patients.

References

1. Hall H. Effective spine triage: patterns of pain. *Ochsner J.* 2014;14(1):88–95. Medline:24688339

2. Hall H, editor. Rheumatology. Boston: MTP Press; c1983. (Harden R, Marcus A, editors. The new medicine: an integrated system of study; vol. 1). http://dx.doi.org/10.1007/978-94-010-9747-5.

3. Sieper J, Rudwaleit M, Baraliakos X, et al. The Assessment of Spondylarthritis International Society (ASAS) handbook: a guide to assess spondylarthritis. *Ann Rheum Dis.* 2009;68(Suppl 2):ii1–44. http://dx.doi.org/10.1136/ard.2008.104018. Medline:19433414

Further Reading

Assessment of Spondylarthritis International Society [Internet]. asas-group.org v.2.2; c2003-2014 [updated 2014 Oct 7]. Available from: http://www.asas-group.org

Chou R, Qaseem A, Snow V, et al; Clinical Efficacy Assessment Subcommittee of the American College of Physicians, and the American College of Physicians; American Pain Society Low Back Pain Guidelines Panel. Diagnosis and treatment of low back pain: a joint clinical practice guideline from the American College of Physicians and the American Pain Society. *Ann Intern Med.* 2007;147(7):478–91. http://dx.doi.org/10.7326/0003-4819-147-7-200710020-00006. Medline:17909209

Fourney DR, Andersson G, Arnold PM, et al. Chronic low back pain: a heterogeneous condition with challenges for an evidence-based approach. *Spine.* 2011;36(21 Suppl):S1–9. http://dx.doi.org/10.1097/BRS.0b013e31822f0a0d. Medline:21952181

9

The Patient at Risk for a Fragility Fracture

DR. HEATHER MCDONALD-BLUMER
UNIVERSITY OF TORONTO

The clinical outcome of concern with osteoporosis is the occurrence of low-trauma fractures, which carry with them a significant morbidity and mortality. Although it is uncommon for patients to be admitted to an acute care hospital with a presenting complaint of osteoporosis, older patients with slip-and-fall injuries causing fracture must be evaluated for osteoporosis either during their hospital stay or shortly thereafter. For those physicians practising in ambulatory settings, the recognition and potential care for patients with or at risk of osteoporosis must be "on your radar screen."

KEY CONCEPTS

Osteoporosis is defined as follows:

- a skeletal disorder characterized by compromised bone strength predisposing a person to fractures (where bone strength reflects the integration of 2 main features: bone density and bone quality)
- a bone density T-score less than or equal to −2.5 (using World Health Organization diagnostic criteria, which are based on a reference population of Caucasian, postmenopausal women)
- the occurrence of 1 or more low-trauma fractures

The diagnosis of osteoporosis is made by assessing the information obtained from the patient's history and physical examination, and from reviewing radiographic studies such as thoracolumbar spine X-rays and dual energy X-ray absorptiometry. Clues to secondary causes may be ascertained from these assessments, but frequently require specific laboratory studies for appropriate evaluation and diagnosis.

- Assessment of risk factors is important in male and female patients from age 50 onward.
- Treatment strategies are guided by 10-year fracture risk assessment, which combines gender, selected clinical risk factors, and bone density data to predict an absolute fracture probability over time.
- Preventive strategies of proper calcium, vitamin D, exercise, and low-risk lifestyle should be encouraged to try to maintain optimal bone health in all at-risk populations.
- Pharmacologic intervention should be strongly considered in those individuals at high risk of an osteoporosis-related fracture.
- Osteoporosis management strategies must be reevaluated at regular intervals to provide optimal patient care.

History

PATIENT DEMOGRAPHICS

Age: Patients over the age of 65 are known to be at higher risk for fracture. Lower age does not exclude a diagnosis of osteoporosis. Risk factor assessment is important—see the next section: "Key Questions."

Gender: Women have a higher risk for low bone density and fractures than men. One in 4 women and 1 in 8 men over the age of 50 have osteoporosis.

Ethnicity: People of Caucasian and Asian descent tend to be at higher risk than people of African descent.

KEY QUESTIONS

With the history, you should be able to determine risk factors for osteoporosis and the impact to date of low bone density (see "2010 Clinical Practice Guidelines for the Diagnosis and Management of Osteoporosis in Canada: Summary"[1]). Ask about **risk factors for fracture**, as these are highly correlated with increased risk of subsequent fracture.

1. What is your age?

Age 65 and older is associated with higher risk for fracture.

2. Have you ever had a minimal-trauma fracture?

- Also known as a fragility or osteoporotic fracture, a minimal-trauma fracture occurs with little or no trauma, such as a fall from standing height.

- Most important are those fractures that occur after the age of 40.

- Axial fractures may present with the sudden onset of localized back pain (about one-third of patients), but two-thirds are clinically silent initially.

- **Inquire about a history of height loss over time:** documented loss of more than 2 cm over time may indicate silent axial fractures and should prompt investigation.

- Pelvic and rib fractures can indicate osteoporosis if they are sustained with minimal trauma.

- Peripheral fracture sites of concern include:
  - wrist (Colle fracture)
  - hip
  - proximal humerus

- Exclusions (fractures that are not considered fragility fractures and do not confer increased risk of subsequent osteoporosis-related fracture) include:

- craniofacial fractures
- metacarpal and metatarsal fractures
- ankle fractures (most—it is important to identify the mechanism of injury)

3. Have you used any glucocorticoids or other high-risk medications?

Inquire about:

- glucocorticoids taken for more than 3 months at doses higher than or equal to 7.5 mg/day
  - See "American College of Rheumatology 2010 Recommendations for the Prevention and Treatment of Glucocorticoid-Induced Osteoporosis."[2]
- anticonvulsants (chronic)
- heparin therapy (chronic)
- hormone suppressive medication: antiestrogen and antiandrogen therapies
- selective serotonin reuptake inhibitors (SSRIs)
- proton pump inhibitors (PPIs)

Also ask about medications that can positively affect bone mass:

- hormonal preparations: estrogens, testosterones, etc.
- osteoporosis therapies:
  - calcium, vitamin D
  - antiresorptive therapies (see below)
- naturopathic therapies (usually of unknown influence on bone)

4. Is there a family history of osteoporosis?

- Osteoporotic fractures in either parent are relevant, although maternal hip fracture carries the highest risk of low bone mass and fragility fracture.

Osteoporosis

- Ask about low bone mass.
- Ask about other illnesses that may be relevant.

• Be on the lookout for unusual histories that might suggest other metabolic bone diseases (e.g., osteogenesis imperfecta).

5. Is there known low bone density?

T-scores less than or equal to -2.5 indicate low bone density. The patient may know about previous dual-energy X-ray absorptiometry (DXA) results, or this could be obtained from the laboratory where it was performed.

6. What is the social history?

Lifestyle factors can influence the attainment of peak bone mass and subsequent maintenance of bone density. The following can be risk factors for osteoporosis and related fractures:

• low calcium intake

• tobacco use

• excess alcohol intake

• excess caffeine intake

• inactivity

• increased risk of falls (due to disorders of sight, mobility, balance, etc.)

7. Are there other medical conditions that could be secondary causes of bone loss?

Assessing the patient for secondary causes of bone loss can be accomplished in part through history taking and physical examination, although supporting investigations are usually needed for an accurate diagnosis. Consider the following:

• **Hormonal insufficiency:**
  - **Women:** Check for late menarche, early menopause, prolonged amenorrhea.
  - **Men:** Check for testosterone deficiency.

   - Also consider diseases and drugs that may interfere with normal hormonal function (see question 3, above, about medications).

- **Malabsorption/malnutrition:** Check for:
  - inappropriately low body weight (hormonal and nutritional roles)
  - loss of more than 10% of usual adult body weight
  - inflammatory bowel disease (Crohn disease and ulcerative colitis)
  - celiac disease
  - post-GI surgery with significant resection

- **Selected other chronic illnesses:** Check for:
  - chronic kidney disease with abnormal creatinine
  - clinical hyperthyroidism
  - rheumatoid arthritis
  - parathyroid disorders
  - malignancy (including multiple myeloma, which can present with low axial bone mineral density or a vertebral fracture)

- **Malignancy** can affect the skeleton directly through the disease process, through subsequent cachexia of malignancy, and through some of the pharmacologic agents used to treat the underlying cancer. Most of this will be evident on the history or physical examination. **Multiple myeloma** can present as "osteoporosis" occasionally.

- **Chronic kidney disease** is usually associated with complex metabolic bone disease, but osteoporosis can occur. When renal impairment is present, creatinine clearance is important for determining the safe use of bisphosphonates (contraindicated for patients with creatinine clearance less than 30–35 mL/m).

- **Impairment of sight** is a risk factor for falling that can lead to increased fracture risk. **Impairment of mobility and balance** carry similar risks. Falls cause fractures even when the bone density is normal, but when an increased risk of falling is combined with low bone density, the resultant risk of fragility fracture is markedly elevated.

8. Is there any additional history regarding osteoporosis?

Inquire about:

- previous investigations
- treatments to date
- activities of daily living

Physical Examination

The general examination is helpful in ruling in or out secondary causes of decreased bone density. The following list describes key points to assess and document in the context of osteoporosis.

Weight: Significant findings include weight of less than 60 kg **or** loss of more than 10% usual adult body weight **or** a body mass index of less than 19 g/m².

Height:

- If previous height measurements are available, loss of more than 2 cm is suggestive of a new vertebral fracture.
- If "recalled" height is all that is available, loss of 4 cm (some sources say 6 cm) is likely significant.
  - The presence of lower limb pathological changes or a severe scoliosis decreases the usefulness of these guidelines.

Kyphosis:
- Use "eyeball" evaluation.

- Kyphosis can be measured more precisely by a kyphometer, but this is generally limited to research.

Focal spinal tenderness: This may suggest an axial fracture.

Occiput-to-wall distance: This should be 0. It increases in setting of vertebral fracture(s).

Rib-to-pelvis distance (measured in midaxillary line):

- Normal distance is more than 2 fingerbreadths.
- This measurement decreases with lower thoracic and lumbar compression fracture.

Gait/balance:

- Look for steady gait, and good balance with standing and position change.
- Poor gait and balance increase risk of falling and subsequent fracture.

Eyesight: Poor vision may be a risk factor for falling.

Key Laboratory Investigations

INITIAL INVESTIGATIONS

CBC: Use this to assess general health status and to screen for nutritional status (e.g., elevated mean corpuscular volume with folate deficiency can occur in the setting of malabsorption disease).

Calcium, phosphate, albumin:

- If elevated calcium, think laboratory error (if a single sample); consider parathyroid disease, malignancy (other less common causes).
- If low calcium, consider chronic illness with low albumin or hypoparathyroidism (multiple causes).
- If vitamin D deficiency, consider dietary deficiencies, malabsorption diseases, liver disease, or renal disease.

Creatinine: If elevated, consider other metabolic bone diseases; monitor vitamin D status. Elevated creatine may affect choice of pharmacologic agents.

Alkaline phosphatase:

- This should be normal in osteoporosis.
- If elevated, consider compression fracture; assess for lytic and/or osteoclastic disease.
- If very low, assess for metabolic bone disease such as hypophosphatasia.

Protein electrophoresis: If elevated, consider monoclonal gammopathy; rule out multiple myeloma.

Erythrocyte sedimentation rate: Use this in older patients to assess for multiple myeloma.

FURTHER CONSIDERATIONS

- Assessment for secondary causes of bone loss is often prompted by the occurrence of a significant nontraumatic fracture history, a dramatic family history of fractures, abnormal results of screening laboratory work, or the presence of unexpectedly low bone density on DXA testing. **Note:** If the Z-score is more than 2.0 standard deviations (SD) below the mean, a diligent search for secondary causes of osteoporosis should be undertaken.

- If the clinical index of suspicion is high or the results of initial screening tests are abnormal, consider the following tests:
  - parathyroid hormone (PTH) (intact)
  - vitamin D (25 hydroxy vitamin D or rarely, 1,25 dihydroxy vitamin D)
  - creatinine clearance
  - immunoelectrophoresis
  - 24-hour urine for calcium excretion

- luteinizing hormone (LH), follicle-stimulating hormone (FSH)
- free or bioavailable testosterone levels
- thyroid-stimulating hormone (TSH)

Imaging

Thoracolumbar spine lateral radiographs:

- These are very useful in assessing patients for vertebral fractures.
- Significant loss of vertebral height is defined as greater than 20% reduction in height when compared with a similar region of an adjacent vertebrae or when compared with the height of intact vertical regions of the same vertebra (anterior height loss often occurs first).
- It may take 3 to 6 weeks for compression to be visible on plain X-ray.

Technetium bone scan:

- This could be considered if you are suspicious of new vertebral fracture and plain radiographs are unrevealing.
- Early fractures take time to reveal compression, whereas the bone scan will usually be positive almost immediately after the fracture has occurred.
- Alternative assessments include CT scan and MRI, depending on their availability.

Dual energy X-ray absorptiometry (DXA):

- This is currently the best quantitative measure of bone mass.
- Low bone density as determined by this technology correlates well with increased occurrence of fragility fracture, especially in older patients.
- DXA may also be useful in monitoring response to treatment over time.

Osteoporosis

- To determine when to order a DXA, use the following criteria:
  - **49 years old and younger:** Reserve for those with major risk factors (e.g., monitoring prolonged corticosteroid use).
  - **50–64 years old:** Consider for those with 2 or more clinical risk factors.
  - **65 years and older:** Do once and repeat, depending on clinical circumstances and baseline test results.
  - **All individuals:** Use to monitor therapy, but do not repeat annually in this setting.

WORLD HEALTH ORGANIZATION DIAGNOSTIC CRITERIA FOR CATEGORIZING BONE MINERAL DENSITY ACCORDING TO DXA

Normal: T-score from −1.0 to +2.5 SD around the mean

Low bone density: T-score from 1.1 to 2.5 SD below the mean (−1.1 to −2.5 SD)

Osteoporosis: T-score less than 2.5 SD below the mean (less than −2.5 SD)

Remember that:

- The "mean" referred to by the T-score is based on young, healthy adults and is sex matched.
- Z-scores may also be given in DXA data:
  - Z-scores compare bone mass to the individual's age-matched controls or peer population.
  - Low Z-scores (Z-score greater than 2 SD below the age-matched mean) suggest a higher probability of secondary causes of low bone density.

Ten-Year Fracture Prediction

CAROC and **FRAX** can both be used to predict 10-year absolute fracture risk.

These fracture-prediction models use age, sex, personal history of low-trauma fracture, and current use of corticosteroids as the key clinical risk factors for calculating the likelihood of an osteoporosis-related fracture over the ensuing 10-year interval.

- FRAX addresses additional risk factors, including family history of an osteoporosis-related fracture and known secondary causes of osteoporosis.

- CAROC requires bone mineral density data; FRAX can calculate 10-year fracture risk with and without these data.

- It is important to remember that the 10-year risk models predict risk of fracture in **treatment-naive individuals.**

- With either model, predicted fracture risk can be helpful in planning treatment (see Table 9.1).

Treatment Options

See Table 9.1 for an overview of treatment options for fragility fracture.

NONPHARMACOLOGIC INTERVENTION

These include:

- appropriate exercise
- fall-prevention strategies
- hip protectors in suitable candidates
- nutritional strategies:
  - adequate calcium intake (preferred delivery is by diet, but include calcium supplementation as required): 1200 mg/day in total, divided throughout the day
  - vitamin D supplementation (men and women):
    - **Individuals with or at risk of osteoporosis** should have vitamin D_3 800–2000 units per day.
    - **Individuals age 50 and older** should have vitamin D_3 800–2000 units/day.
    - **Healthy individuals age 18 to 49** should have vitamin D_3 400 units/day.

TABLE 9.1. Overview of treatment approach based on 10-year fracture risk

10-year fracture risk	Treatment approach
Low risk	
10-year fracture risk estimated to be < 10%	Lifestyle modification Amelioration of risk factors
High risk*	
10-year fracture risk estimated to be > 20%	Lifestyle modification Amelioration of risk factors Pharmacologic treatment (should be considered)
Moderate risk	
10-year fracture risk estimated to be between 10% and 20%	Lifestyle modification Amelioration of risk factors Pharmacologic treatment (should be considered): The clinician must assess the patient fully (fall risk, general health, family history, patient preferences, etc.) when determining which individuals in the moderate-risk group may benefit from pharmacologic therapy. For example, a moderate-risk individual who has mobility issues and falls frequently could benefit from the addition of an antiresorptive agent to minimize fracture risk, whereas an individual of the same age and bone mineral density who is completely well and does not have a risk of falls could be well managed conservatively.

*FRAX defines high risk as calculated hip fracture risk > 3% or any osteoporotic fracture risk of > 20%.

PHARMACOLOGIC MEASURES

- A review of the "2010 Clinical Practice Guidelines for the Diagnosis and Management of Osteoporosis in Canada: Summary"[1] is strongly recommended for a summary of the current evidenced-based recommendations.

- The use of bone-modifying medication in the management of osteoporosis is similar to the use of all medications and must be predicated on an assessment of the potential benefit outweighing the potential harm. Periodic reassessment of the benefit-to-risk balance is recommended, as all current pharmacologic therapies used in the management of osteoporosis have potential side effects and risks that must be considered when planning treatment.

- The recent recognition of horizontal atraumatic subtrochanteric fractures in a very small proportion of patients who have low bone density and have been treated with antiresorptive drugs has raised concern regarding the long-term safety of these medications, bisphosphonates in particular.

  - Although a cause-effect relationship has not been established, there is concern that long-term exposure to these medications can inhibit bone repair and lead to the development of "chalk stick" or atypical femur fractures.
  - Routine assessment regarding the ongoing need of these drug therapies is recommended, in addition to screening questions regarding updated fracture history, duration of use of medication, and presence of possible symptoms of incomplete femur fracture such as bilateral proximal anterolateral thigh pain.
  - When concern is present, consideration should be given to obtaining plain X-rays, which can be helpful in looking for early radiographic changes heralding these fractures.
  - In addition, technetium bone scans, CT, or MRI can be considered.
  - Referral to an expert in osteoporosis care and/or an orthopedic surgeon is recommended for individuals with clinical or radiographic features suggesting an atypical femur fracture.

Osteoporosis

- Patients who are not at high risk of an osteoporotic fracture should generally not remain on these therapies unless there are specific concerns regarding falls and elevated fracture risk.
- Consideration of a "drug holiday" is controversial and warrants careful weighing of the pros and cons for each patient.

ANTIRESORPTIVE AGENTS

Oral bisphosphonates

Options and doses are as follows:

- alendronate (multiple generic versions):
  - Fosamax 10 mg orally once daily or 70 mg orally once weekly
  - Fosavance 70 mg of alendronate weekly, and either 2800 or 5600 units of vitamin D weekly
- risedronate (multiple generic versions):
  - Actonel 5 mg orally once daily, 35 mg orally once weekly, or 150 mg orally once monthly
  - Actonel DR 35 mg orally once weekly at the end of a breakfast meal

Comments

Oral bisphosphonates:

- have strong data to support fracture reduction (axial and peripheral-hip) in the patient with osteoporosis
- are effective in minimizing glucocorticoid-induced osteoporosis (GIOP) and related fractures
- are appropriate for use in women and men
- have a specific protocol to minimize esophageal irritation
- are contraindicated in those with creatinine clearance less than 30 mL/min

- may carry risk of atypical femoral fracture with prolonged treatment
- are poorly absorbed: have crucial dosing instructions
- require adequate calcium and vitamin D intake (crucial to emphasize)

Intravenous bisphosphonate
The option is zoledronate (e.g., Aclasta) 5 mg IV **once** yearly.

Comments
Intravenous bisphosphonate:

- has strong data to support fracture reduction (axial and peripheral hip) in the osteoporotic patient
- has no concerns regarding GI side effects
- carries renal cautions (acute renal dysfunction has been reported rarely)
- is contraindicated in those with creatinine clearance less than 35 mL/min
- may carry risk of atypical femoral fracture with prolonged use
- requires adequate calcium and vitamin D intake (crucial to emphasize)

RANK ligand inhibitor
The option is denosumab: Prolia 60 mg subcutaneously every 6 months.

Comments
RANK ligand inhibitor:

- has strong data to support antifracture benefits (axial and peripheral)
- has a potential advantage in adherence
- can be used in moderate renal dysfunction
- carries risk of atypical femoral fracture with prolonged use

Osteoporosis

Selective estrogen receptor modulator (SERM)

The option is raloxifene: Evista 60 mg orally once daily.

Comments

SERM:

- is effective in reducing axial fractures in postmenopausal women
- has no published prospective hip data
- can exacerbate hot flashes
- carries slightly increased risk of venous thrombotic events

Hormone replacement (HR)

Estrogen

- Although estrogen has been shown to minimize osteoporotic fractures in postmenopausal women, the side-effect profile is considerable and the use of estrogen is generally not recommended for the management of osteoporosis.

Testosterone

- In the male population, the use of testosterone may be helpful in selected circumstances when testosterone deficiency has been documented clearly.
- Routine use in the management of male osteoporosis does not appear appropriate.

ANABOLIC AGENT

Parathyroid hormone analogue

The option is teriparatide: Forteo 20 μg subcutaneously daily for maximum course of 24 months.

Comments

Parathyroid hormone analogue:

- is a potent anabolic agent

- is used for severe osteoporosis
- increases risk for osteosarcoma: therefore **not** for use in pediatric patients, the setting of malignancy where there is a risk of bone metastases, Paget disease, prior skeletal radiation, increased alkaline phosphatase

PEARLS

1. In the adult population, all **fragility fractures** carry an increased risk of subsequent fragility fracture. Investigation and treatment are to be strongly considered.

2. All patients starting prolonged **glucocorticoid therapy** must be considered at high risk for osteoporosis and its consequences—specifically vertebral fracture. This can occur within the first year of steroid therapy, particularly in those taking high-dose steroids or in those already at risk for osteoporosis/fractures.

   For individuals taking prednisone 7.5 mg/day or more for 3 or more months, suitable treatment is required:

   a. Optimize calcium and vitamin D intake.

   b. Counsel patients regarding suitable lifestyle habits (tobacco avoidance, minimal alcohol and caffeine, exercise as able, etc.).

   c. Conduct DXA testing as baseline.

   d. Conduct DXA testing 12 months after institution of corticosteroids (and bone protective management).

   e. Establish bone markers.

   f. Consider use of either a bisphosphonate or denosumab as a preventative or therapeutic strategy (see "American College of Rheumatology 2010 Recommendations for the Prevention and Treatment of Glucocorticoid-Induced Osteoporosis"[2]).

3. **Z-score of −2.0 or lower** indicates that bone density is low for an individual's age and, as such, suitable investigation is required.

Osteoporosis

References

1. Papaioannou A, Morin S, Cheung AM, et al; Scientific Advisory Council of Osteoporosis Canada. 2010 clinical practice guidelines for the diagnosis and management of osteoporosis in Canada: summary. *CMAJ*. 2010;182(17):1864–73. http://dx.doi.org/10.1503/cmaj.100771. Medline:20940232

2. Grossman JM, Gordon R, Ranganath VK, et al. American College of Rheumatology 2010 recommendations for the prevention and treatment of glucocorticoid-induced osteoporosis. *Arthritis Care Res (Hoboken)*. 2010;62(11):1515–26. http://dx.doi.org/10.1002/acr.20295. Medline:20662044

Further Reading

Brown JP, Morin S, Leslie W, et al. Bisphosphonates for treatment of osteoporosis: expected benefits, potential harms, and drug holidays. *Can Fam Physician*. 2014;60(4):324–33. Medline:24733321

Green AD, Colón-Emeric CS, Bastian L, et al. Does this woman have osteoporosis? *JAMA*. 2004;292(23):2890–900. http://dx.doi.org/10.1001/jama.292.23.2890. Medline:15598921

International Society for Clinical Densitometry. 2013 ISCD official positions – adult [Internet]. cISCD; 2013 Aug [updated 2013 Aug 15; modified 2014 Apr 24; cited 2014 Dec 5]. Available from: http://www.iscd.org/official-positions/2013-iscd-official-positions-adult/

Osteoporosis prevention, diagnosis, and therapy. NIH consensus statement online [Internet]. 2000 March 27–29 [cited 2014 June]; 17(1): 1–36. Available from: http://consensus.nih.gov/2000/2000osteoporosis111html.htm

Shane, Burr D, Abrahamsen B, et al. Atypical subtrochanteric and diaphyseal femoral fractures: second report of a task force of the American College for Bone and Mineral Research. *J Bone Miner Res*. 2014;29(1):1–23. http://dx.doi.org/10.1002/jbmr.1998. Medline:23712442

SECTION 2: APPROACH TO THE SELECTION AND INTERPRETATION OF INVESTIGATIONS IN THE MANAGEMENT OF RHEUMATIC DISEASES

10

Selection and Interpretation of Laboratory Investigations

DR. MAX SUN AND DR. KAM SHOJANIA
UNIVERSITY OF BRITISH COLUMBIA

KEY CONCEPTS

There are 3 reasons to order laboratory investigations in rheumatology:

- to confirm a diagnosis or determine the extent of a disease—e.g., antinuclear antibodies (ANAs) in systemic lupus erythematosus (SLE)
- to monitor disease activity—e.g., ESR in giant cell arteritis or anti-double-stranded DNA (anti-dsDNA) in SLE
- to monitor drug toxicity—e.g., transaminase monitoring when using methotrexate

Laboratory investigations are useful only as an adjunct to a thorough history and physical examination and can only be interpreted in the context of a specific clinical situation. A good clinician will be wary of putting too much emphasis on the laboratory. In general, a diagnostic investigation is most helpful when the sensitivity and specificity are high, and when the pretest probability of the condition is question is about 50%.

Determining the usefulness of lab tests

To determine the usefulness of a test in a specific situation, you need to know 2 things:

- the intrinsic qualities of the test, which are constant and include:
  - sensitivity (the proportion of patients with the disease that have a positive test)
  - specificity (the proportion of patients without the disease that have a negative test)
- the pretest probability of disease (the likelihood of disease in a particular situation), which is obtained by thorough history taking and physical examination, and by interpretation of other supporting investigations (X-rays, ECG, ultrasound, etc.)

PRETEST AND POSTTEST PROBABILITY

For **pretest probability**, the clinician estimates the likelihood of the disease **before** the test is performed.

The clinician can calculate **posttest probability,** using Bayes' theorem, with the following formula:

Posttest probability if the test is positive:

$$\frac{100}{1 + \left\{ \dfrac{100 - \text{Pretest Probability}}{\text{Pretest Probability}} \right\} \left\{ \dfrac{100 - \text{Specificity}}{\text{Sensitivity}} \right\}}$$

Posttest probability if the test is negative:

$$\frac{100}{1 + \left\{ \dfrac{100 - \text{Pretest Probability}}{\text{Pretest Probability}} \right\} \left\{ \dfrac{\text{Specificity}}{100 - \text{Sensitivity}} \right\}}$$

Example calculation of posttest probability

Let's use the example of HLA-B27. In a Caucasian patient, the sensitivity is 92% and the specificity is 92% for ankylosing spondylitis. After examining the patient, you decide that your pretest probability that the patient has ankylosing spondylitis is 50%.

Application of Bayes' theorem will result in the following posttest probabilities:

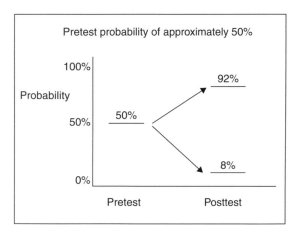

With a pretest probability of 50%, the HLA-B27 test is helpful if the result is positive or negative. However, if your pretest probability of ankylosing spondylitis is very low or very high, the test becomes less helpful. The following graph represents the outcomes of using the HLA-B27 test in 2 patients, 1 with a low pretest probability (10%) and 1 with a high pretest probability (90%):

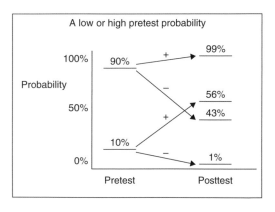

The 50:50 rule

If your pretest likelihood of a disease is about 50%:

- The posttest likelihood that a patient **has** the disease, given a **positive** test result, is approximately equal to **specificity**.

- The posttest likelihood that a patient **does not have** the disease, given a **negative** test result, is approximately equal to **sensitivity**.

Specific laboratory investigations in rheumatology

ESR AND CRP

Description

The ESR is a measure of the rate (mm/hour) at which RBCs settle through a column of plasma. Measuring the ESR takes approximately 1 hour. It is an indirect test of globulins and fibrinogen, which are increased in inflammatory states. Globulins and fibrinogen disrupt the repellent forces between RBCs and allow RBCs to settle at a faster rate (thus producing a higher test value). The ESR is time intensive compared with measurement of CRP, which is an automated test that measures a specific acute phase reactant. CRP is produced by the liver during periods of inflammation and is detectable in the blood serum of patients with various infectious or inflammatory diseases. It is influenced by interleukin-6 levels.

Use

These nonspecific tests are sometimes helpful in distinguishing between inflammatory and noninflammatory conditions. However, they are not diagnostic and may be abnormal in a vast array of infectious, malignant, rheumatic, and other diseases. They can also be within the normal range in the face of active disease (e.g., SLE).

- An ESR above 40 mm/h may indicate polymyalgia rheumatica (PMR) or giant cell arteritis if the patient's history and physical examination are compatible with either diagnosis. Unfortunately, the ESR may be below 40 mm/h in up to 20% of patients with these conditions. A very high CRP or ESR (higher than 100) should prompt consideration of vasculitis, significant infection, or malignancy.

- The ESR and CRP may be useful for monitoring patients with rheumatoid arthritis (RA), PMR, and giant cell arteritis, where a rise may herald a worsening of the disease when a glucocorticoid dose is being tapered. This should not automatically result in an increase in the steroid dose: rather, it should prompt closer observation and perhaps a more gradual tapering of the steroid.

Common pitfalls

- Using the ESR to screen for inflammation is usually not helpful because the sedimentation rate can rise with anemia, infections, and the use of certain medications such as cholesterol-lowering drugs. The ESR also tends to rise with age and is of limited value in the elderly; an elevated ESR in an elderly patient should not prompt further investigation in the absence of clinical findings.
  - A rough rule of thumb for the upper limit for ESR with increasing age is as follows:

ESR, upper limit of normal for men = age/2

ESR, upper limit of normal for women = (age + 10)/2

- The CRP test is more reliable than the ESR, as it does not rise with anemia and rises only slightly with age. The CRP is also now cheaper than the ESR.

- Clinicians still rely on the ESR for some clinical diagnoses such as PMR, but the CRP can be used in this setting to support the finding of an abnormal ESR. Connective tissue diseases (SLE, scleroderma, dermatomyositis) may have modest or absent CRP elevation, although in the setting of superimposed infection, CRP may well be elevated. CRP is produced by the liver, and so liver failure may decrease CRP values. In addition, a major limitation of CRP is its tendency to be a very dynamic protein with fairly wide swings observed from day to day.

RHEUMATOID FACTOR

Description

Rheumatoid factor (RF) is a misnomer: it confers specificity to this test that is not based on clinical evidence. Classic RFs are IgM antibodies directed against the Fc (constant) region of the IgG molecule. Their presence can be detected with a wide variety of techniques—e.g., latex particles coated with human IgG, enzyme-linked immunosorbent assay (ELISA), or nephelometry. Unfortunately, there is no universal interlaboratory standardization for the measurement of RF. Rheumatoid factor is present in most people at very low levels, but higher levels are present in 5% to 10% of the population, and this percentage rises with age.

Use

- Many conditions can cause elevated RF (see Table 10.1).

TABLE 10.1. Some conditions associated with an abnormal rheumatoid factor (RF)

Rheumatologic diseases	Other conditions
Rheumatoid arthritis	Cryoglobulinemia (RF can act as a surrogate marker)
Sjögren syndrome	
Systemic sclerosis	Endocarditis
Idiopathic inflammatory myopathies (polymyositis/dermatomyositis)	Mycobacterial diseases
	Viral hepatitis
Mixed connective tissue disease	Syphilis
Sarcoidosis	Advanced age (RF can be adjusted for age)
Systemic lupus erythematosus	

- Only about 60% of patients with RA test above the normal range for RF, with specificity of approximately 80%. However, in patients with RA, a high-titre test may predict a more severe disease course and increased extra-articular manifestations.
- This test should be done only if a patient is suspected to have RA or Sjögren syndrome.
- Serial testing is not useful for patients with RA or any other condition.
- In patients with RA who have failed conventional disease-modifying antirheumatic drugs and are being treated with biologic agents, RF positivity has been reported to predict a better response to rituximab.

Common pitfalls
- Rheumatoid factor is not useful as a screening test.
- It is nonspecific and insensitive: the presence of RF does not necessarily indicate a diagnosis of RA, nor does its absence rule out the disease. The finding of positive RF in a patient with nonspecific symptoms should not precipitate

unnecessary investigations. However, recent studies have shown that asymptomatic patients with positive RF results may be at higher risk for developing RA in the future.

ANTICITRULLINATED PROTEIN ANTIBODIES

Description

Anticitrullinated protein antibodies (ACPAs) are IgG antibodies that bind to proteins that have undergone posttranslational changes during inflammation (replacement of the amino acid arginine with citrulline). These antibodies have high affinity for epitopes containing citrulline. Commercial assays use ELISA and bead-based immunoassays to detect ACPAs that recognize a variety of synthetic citrullinated peptides as antigens. These are collectively referred to as anti-cyclic citrullinated peptide (anti-CCP) antibodies. ACPAs are specific for RA (95 to 96%), with a sensitivity of approximately 70% to 75%.

Use

- The presence of ACPAs has been shown to correlate with increased disease severity and increased risk of radiographic progression of joint damage.
- ACPAs are highly specific for RA, and they have also been found in other diseases such as SLE, primary Sjögren syndrome, tuberculosis, hepatitis C infections, other infectious diseases, and malignancies.
- ACPAs have been implicated as a risk factor for the development of RA, with several studies showing the presence of ACPAs in asymptomatic patients before disease diagnosis.
- They can become positive years before RF is elevated:

- Twenty percent of RF-negative patients are positive for ACPA.
- The positive predictive value for development of RA in a patient positive for **both** RF and anti-CCP is close to 100%.

- ACPAs are often requested in combination with RF, and can help confirm RA in individuals with undifferentiated polyarthritis. They are also a helpful prognostic factor for severe disease.

Common pitfalls
ACPA levels do not change with disease activity and should not be used to adjust therapy.

ANTINUCLEAR ANTIBODIES

Description
Antinuclear antibodies are a diverse group of autoantibodies that bind to the proteins or nucleic acids within the cell nucleus, although contemporary terminology includes autoantibodies that bind to some cytoplasmic antigens as well. There are multiple subtypes of ANAs and each binds to a different macromolecular complex. Some have specific disease associations.

There are many assays to detect ANA. The most sensitive is the indirect immunofluorescence (IIF) assay based on HEp-2 cells as the substrate for antibody binding.

Many autoimmune diseases are associated with ANA positivity. There are also many other conditions associated with positive ANA results (see Table 10.2). ANA is positive in 98% of patients with SLE, 40% to 70% of those with other connective tissue diseases, up to 20% of those with autoimmune thyroid and liver disease, and in 5% of healthy adults (at a cut-off titre of 1:160). A negative ANA result virtually rules out SLE because of high sensitivity of ANA tests.

TABLE 10.2. Some conditions associated with positive ANA

Rheumatologic disease	Other conditions
Systemic lupus erythematosus (SLE)	Autoimmune liver disease (autoimmune hepatitis, primary biliary cirrhosis)
Mixed connective tissue disease	
Scleroderma	Autoimmune thyroid disease
Sjögren syndrome	Healthy relatives of SLE patients
	Neoplasia
	Advanced age

Abbreviation: ANA, antinuclear antibody.

TABLE 10.3. Common patterns of antinuclear antibodies

Pattern	Association	Further tests suggested
Speckled	Nonspecific	Test for extractable nuclear antigens (may be helpful)
Homogeneous	Nonspecific	Test for anti-dsDNA, histones, and/or chromatin
Nucleolar	Diffuse scleroderma	Test for anti-topoisomerase antibodies (may be helpful)
Centromere	Limited scleroderma (CREST)	None
Rim	SLE (anti-dsDNA)	Anti-dsDNA

Abbreviations: anti-dsDNA, anti-double-stranded DNA; CREST, *c*alcinosis, *R*aynaud phenomenon, *e*sophageal dysmotility, *s*clerodactyly, *t*elangiectasias; SLE, systemic lupus erythematosus.

Results are typically reported as a titre (serial dilutions of samples are each tested for response, and the highest dilution that still gives a positive test is reported) with a pattern (Table 10.3), which is occasionally useful in making a diagnosis of a connective tissue disease. However, it is now recognized that many of these staining patterns have low sensitivity and specificity. One notable exception is the anticentromere pattern, which is specific for limited scleroderma (CREST syndrome). There are several different ways to detect ANAs.

Use

- Testing for ANA should be ordered when a connective tissue disease such as SLE is suspected on the basis of several specific findings on history and/or physical examination (see chapter 5b). These findings could include photosensitivity, malar rash, alopecia, mouth ulcers, sicca symptoms, Raynaud phenomenon, inflammatory arthritis, pleuropericarditis, or glomerulonephritis.
- If the test is negative, SLE can usually be ruled out.
- A positive test result does not by itself confirm a diagnosis of connective tissue disease.
- Serial testing is usually of no value, as ANA does not accurately reflect disease activity.

Common pitfalls

At a cut-off titre of 1:40, a staggering 32% of the normal population is positive for ANA (13% is positive at a titre of 1:80). Since only 0.1% of the population has SLE, **a low-titre ANA result is almost always of no consequence. If history and physical examination are unremarkable, no further investigation of a positive ANA should be done.**

TESTS FOR ANTIBODIES TO EXTRACTABLE NUCLEAR ANTIGENS

Description

An extractable nuclear antigen (ENA) panel tests for specific antibodies to nuclear and cytoplasmic antigens obtained from a variety of sources. There are a large number of ENAs, but most are used for research purposes. ENAs that are commercially available include anti-SSB/La, anti-SSA/Ro60, anti-Smith (Sm), anti-U1RNP, anti-Scl-70 (topoisomerase I), anti-chromatin/nucleosome, anti-ribosomal P, and anti-Jo-1.

Use

- A test for antibodies to ENAs (anti-ENA) should be ordered only if there is a suspected or known connective tissue disease and the ANA test result is positive at a significant titre (1:160 or higher).
- Many positive anti-ENA results can point to a specific connective tissue disease (see (Table 10.4).

TABLE 10.4. Rheumatic disease associations with antibodies against specific extractable nuclear antigens

Antibodies to specific extractable nuclear antigens	Rheumatic disease associations
anti-Sm	This is highly specific for SLE, but has low sensitivity
anti-Ro60 (SSA)	This occurs in SLE, especially with cutaneous involvement, and is common in Sjögren syndrome
	Antibodies in the mother are associated with neonatal SLE, including congenital heart block
anti-La (SSB)	This occurs in Sjögren syndrome and SLE
anti-U1RNP	This is nonspecific, but is part of the criteria for MCTD
	It also occurs in SLE
anti-Jo-1	This is highly specific for a severe form of PM/DM, but it is not sensitive
anti-chromatin/-nucleosome	This is seen in SLE and drug-induced SLE
anticentromere	This is typically found in limited scleroderma (CREST)
anti-topoisomerase I (Scl-70)	This is typically found in diffuse scleroderma
	It can correlate with interstitial lung disease
anti-ribosomal P	This is specific for SLE
	It is associated with early onset neuropsychiatric lupus

Abbreviations: CREST, calcinosis, *Raynaud* phenomenon, *e*sophageal dysmotility, *s*clerodactyly, *t*elangiectasias; DM, dermatomyositis; MCTD, mixed connective tissue disease; PM, polymyositis; SLE, systemic lupus erythematosus.

Lab Investigations

- Some positive anti-ENA results indicate the possibility of more severe disease manifestations: for example, the presence of anti-Jo-1 antibody in the setting of inflammatory myopathies often predicts an aggressive course of the disease with interstitial lung disease and inflammatory arthritis.

Common pitfalls

- There are no major pitfalls, although testing is rarely needed (generally not required by the primary care physician).
- Most anti-ENA tests have low or moderate sensitivity, so negative test results are usually not helpful. An exception would be a negative anti-Ro or anti-La result in a pregnant patient with SLE, which may predict a smaller chance of having a child with neonatal lupus.

TEST FOR ANTI-dsDNA ANTIBODY

Description

Antibodies to DNA can be divided into 2 groups:

- those that react to denatured or single-stranded DNA (ssDNA)
- those that recognize double-stranded DNA (dsDNA)

Tests for anti-ssDNA have limited usefulness and are not generally available. In contrast, anti-dsDNA antibodies are relatively specific (95%) for SLE, making them useful for diagnosis, although a negative test result does not rule out the disease, as anti-dsDNA antibody is present in only about 60% of patients with SLE.

Use

- This test should be ordered only when SLE is suspected after clinical evaluation has been performed and the ANA test result is positive.

- The presence of anti-dsDNA antibody may predict a more severe form of SLE with renal or CNS involvement.
- Some clinicians suggest that this test may be useful in following the clinical course of SLE, although this is disputed. Most rheumatologists would not treat an isolated rise in the anti-dsDNA level in the absence of a clinical flare.

- There are 4 assays used to detect dsDNA antibodies. It is important to know which technique is being reported, as the sensitivities and specificities are different.
  - **Farr assay:** This uses radioactively labelled dsDNA to pull down anti-dsDNA antibodies. It is positive in approximately 50% to 80% of all SLE patients.
  - **Crithidia luciliae assay:** This is an immunofluorescence assay that has similar sensitivities to the Farr assay, but may have better specificity.
  - **ELISA:** This has similar sensitivity but lower specificity than the other 2 assays.
  - **Fluorescent addressable, antigen-coated beads combined with laser detection of bound dsDNA antibodies:** This is usually part of a multiplex assay. It can have poor sensitivity and specificity.

Common pitfalls
This test should never be performed as part of a routine screening process for patients with nonspecific musculoskeletal symptoms.

COMPLEMENT (C3 AND C4)
Description
Decreased levels of complement are the result of disorders mediated by circulating immune

TABLE 10.5. Some causes of low serum complements

Rheumatic disease	Other diseases
Systemic lupus erythematosus(may have hereditary complement deficiencies)	Subacute bacterial endocarditis
Cryoglobulinemia	Bacterial sepsis
	Viremias
Rheumatoid vasculitis	Parasitemias
Systemic vasculitis (especially polyarteritis nodosa and urticarial vasculitis)	

complexes such as SLE, selected forms of vasculitis (e.g., essential mixed cryoglobulinemia and rheumatoid vasculitis), and certain types of glomerulonephritis (see Table 10.5). Immune complexes activate the complement cascade through the classical pathway, and this activation results in the consumption of C3 and C4 with reduced levels in the blood. There are also inherited deficiencies of complement; C4 deficiency can be associated with SLE.

Use

In some patients with known vasculitis or SLE, complement levels may reflect disease activity.

- It is expected that an SLE flare will result in decreased complement levels because of activation of the classical complement pathway by immune complexes.

- In most cases, the low complements are a result of increased activation that outstrips synthesis, but in a minority of cases, there seems to be decreased liver synthesis of complements altogether.

- An elevated complement level is a nonspecific finding, but complements are acute phase reactants and therefore may be elevated in inflammatory states or pregnancy.

Common pitfalls

- Measurement of serum complements is not a good screening test on its own. In the context of a clinical presentation that suggests lupus, along with other laboratory features, low C3/C4 levels can support the diagnosis of lupus.
- Interpretation of complement levels may be difficult in the setting of severe infection or pregnancy, as levels may rise.

ANTINEUTROPHIL CYTOPLASMIC ANTIBODY (ANCA) TEST

Description

ANCAs are autoantibodies to the cytoplasmic constituents of granulocytes. They are typically first detected by indirect immunofluorescence (IIF) assay on ethanol-fixed neutrophils and produce a characteristic cytoplasmic fluorescence (cANCA) or perinuclear fluorescence (pANCA). They can also be tested by ELISA or bead-based technologies with purified specific antigens. The IIF assay is more sensitive, while the ELISA and bead-based assays are more specific. Thus, you can screen with immunofluorescence and confirm with the ELISA tests. Unfortunately, testing for ANCA can be variable, with large interlaboratory variability, which decreases its sensitivity and specificity.

ANCAs characteristically occur in small vessel vasculitic syndromes such as:

- granulomatosis with polyangiitis (GPA) (previously known as Wegener granulomatosis)
- microscopic polyangiitis (MPA)
- eosinophilic granulomatosis with polyangiitis (EGPA) (previously known as Churg-Strauss syndrome)

The relevant target antigens associated with vasculitis are proteinase 3 (PR3) for cANCA and myeloperoxidase (MPO) for pANCA. PR3 and MPO are proteases found in neutrophil granules.

ANCAs occur in more than 90% of patients with systemic GPA (with renal and/or pulmonary involvement) and 75% of patients with limited GPA (without renal involvement), 70% of patients with MPA, and 50% of patients with EGPA. The presence of PR3-ANCA is 97% specific for GPA. However, be aware that the absence of ANCA does not exclude the diagnosis of GPA. In patients who are positive for cANCA, changes in the level may reflect disease activity but cannot be used reliably to guide treatment.

Perinuclear ANCAs (pANCAs) occur in a wide range of diseases. They are directed against different cytoplasmic constituents of neutrophils, including MPO, lactoferrin, elastase, and other unspecified antigens. Therefore, a positive pANCA result is nonspecific. Only antibodies to MPO have a significant vasculitis association. A small percentage (10% to 15%) of GPA patients are pANCA positive. Approximately 70% of patients with MPA are MPO-ANCA positive. Perinuclear ANCA may also be seen in EGPA.

Use

The cANCA test can be helpful in confirming a diagnosis of GPA, MPA, or idiopathic crescentic glomerulonephritis.

- PR3-ANCA has a high specificity of 98% for these conditions.
- It has a high sensitivity for systemic GPA (with renal involvement), but less sensitivity for the limited condition (upper respiratory tract involvement without renal involvement).

- A positive PR3-ANCA test result in a patient with typical GPA may obviate the need for a tissue biopsy.

The pANCA test is not useful unless it is confirmed by testing for anti-MPO, which may occur in several related diseases: MPA, EGPA, and crescentic glomerulonephritis.

Common pitfalls

- This test helps in the diagnosis and management of only a very small number of patients with relatively rare conditions. A primary care physician will rarely need to order this test.
- Using ANCAs to screen patients with nonspecific symptoms can result in many false-positive tests.
- Immunofluorescence produces pANCAs in patients with immune-mediated conditions such as collagen vascular disease, inflammatory bowel disease (which can also be associated with cANCA), and autoimmune hepatitis. However, these are not true anti-MPO ANCAs and may have other antigen specificities as outlined earlier.
- Up to 40% of patients with limited GPA and 10% of those with severe disease are ANCA negative. In addition, up to 30% of patients with MPA and half of those with EGPA are also ANCA negative. Some patients who were initially ANCA negative can subsequently become ANCA positive. Thus, a negative ANCA result cannot definitively rule out these types of vasculitis if the clinical scenario fits.
- Another form of vasculitis, polyarteritis nodosa, is defined by ANCA **negativity**.
- Patients with vasculitis are positive for either MPO-ANCA or PR3-ANCA, but never both. Dual positivity suggests an alternate diagnosis.

ANTIPHOSPHOLIPID ANTIBODIES

Description

Antiphospholipid (aPL) antibodies are immunoglobulins directed against negatively charged phospholipids or phospholipid-binding serum proteins. The 3 most important and commonly ordered tests are:

- anticardiolipin (aCL) antibodies
- anti-β2 glycoprotein-I (anti-β2GPI) antibodies
- lupus anticoagulant (LAC)

The target proteins include β2GPI (an apolipoprotein that binds to cardiolipin and acts as a natural anticoagulant) and human prothrombin alone or phosphatidylserine-prothrombin complex. Anti-β2GPI antibodies are considered the hallmark of antiphospholipid syndrome (APS) with high specificity. However, aCL antibodies are more sensitive.

Lupus anticoagulant is a misnomer: these are antibodies that prolong phospholipid-dependent coagulation assays, but are associated with paradoxical clotting in vivo. Rather than being measured by ELISA, LAC is detected through a functional assay. These antibodies block prothrombinase complex, thus producing a prolonged coagulation profile in vitro determined by prolonged activated partial thromboplastin time (aPTT), dilute Russell viper venom time (dRVVT), and kaolin clotting time. In addition, there will be a noncorrecting mixing study (50:50 mix with normal plasma to test for clotting factor deficiency), indicating the presence of a coagulation inhibitor in the plasma. Finally, a source of excess phospholipid (such as frozen platelets) is introduced, which should correct the prolonged coagulation assays by overwhelming the antibodies. The antibodies causing LAC activity are distinct subgroups of antibodies directed against β2GPI or prothrombin and have different antigen specificities compared with aCL antibodies.

Antiphospholipid antibodies are usually seen in APS, which can occur as a secondary syndrome in patients with SLE and other connective tissue diseases, or can manifest as a primary syndrome. These antibodies are associated with a thrombotic state, manifesting as venous and/or arterial thrombosis (e.g., deep vein thrombosis, pulmonary embolism, strokes) and recurrent pregnancy morbidity. Thus, the presence of these antibodies has implications for anticoagulation in the secondary prevention of thromboembolism in patients who have aPL antibodies and in obstetrical APS.

Use

According to the 2009 International Society on Thrombosis and Hemostasis/Scientific and Standardization Committee guidelines, the diagnosis of APS requires the combination of at least:

- 1 supporting clinical feature
- 1 persistently positive aPL assay done 12 weeks apart

Recommendations are to use 2 ELISA tests (aCL and aβ2GPI) and 2 assays (aPTT and dRVVT) for LAC detection.

Thus, patients are tested for aPL antibodies in the setting of 1 or more unexplained thromboembolic events, or recurrent unexplained pregnancy loss. Patients with SLE are at particularly high risk for developing aPL antibodies. Thus, patients with SLE should be tested for aPL antibodies at diagnosis. Positive tests can have treatment implications

Lab Investigations

for women with SLE who want to get pregnant, or those with previous recurrent unexplained pregnancy loss.

An IgG aCL titre of over 35 to 40 GPL is associated with increased risk of thrombosis. The aCL ELISA test has a sensitivity of 80% to 90% for APS, and the sensitivity of anti-β2GPI ranges from 40% to 90%. Tests for aCL antibodies include different types of antibodies reactive to multiple epitopes. Antibodies that bind to β2GPI are an independent risk factor for thrombosis and pregnancy morbidity. Patients with positive aCL antibody results but negative anti-β2GPI antibody results may have a significantly lower risk of clotting. LAC has the strongest association with thrombosis, with an odds ratio ranging from 5 to 16 times above LAC-negative controls.

Common pitfalls

- Even though LAC is associated with several abnormal blood tests, only half of patients demonstrate a prolonged aPTT. Thus, if clinical suspicion is high, consider the dRVVT test. Usually both tests are done in the initial workup.

- Patients with any positive aCL antibody results may have a history of false-positive syphilis screening tests such as positive Venereal Disease Research Laboratory (VDRL) and rapid plasma reagin test results. However, these patients will have negative treponemal-specific assay results if the aCL antibodies are due to APS.

- The initial tests for aPL should always be repeated if the results are positive, as transient elevation in aPL antibody levels are common. Note that aCL antibodies can become temporarily positive in infections such as syphilis, Lyme disease, hepatitis C, tuberculosis, HIV, and others, as well as in drug reactions. The test for LAC is laboratory dependent, and studies have shown a 25% false-positive rate among nonspecialized centres, reaffirming the need for repeating the tests.

- While most patients with APS have positive test results for aCL and LAC, 10% to 16% are positive only for LAC and 25% are positive only for aCL. In a small percentage of patients, anti-β2GPI may be the sole antibody-positive result. IgM and IgA aPL antibodies do exist; however, IgG aCL confers the greatest risk of thrombosis compared with IgM and IgA subtypes.

- Anti-β2GPI antibody testing may not be available at all centres, but samples can be shipped to a laboratory that has the appropriate test. In a clinically suspicious patient with low-titre aCL, testing for β2GPI antibodies will be more sensitive. A newer test that detects antibodies to the phosphatidyl serine/prothrombin complex shows promise for replacing the LAC test in the future.

- Some anticoagulants may interfere with assays for LAC. It is prudent to alert the laboratory to any anticoagulants being used by the patient, so that appropriate modifications can be done, if possible. ELISA testing is not affected by patient use of anticoagulants.

SERUM URIC ACID
Use
- This test is helpful in monitoring the extent of hyperuricemia in patients with gout.
- The prevalence of asymptomatic hyperuricemia among men is 5% to 8%, and fewer than 1 in

3 people with hyperuricemia will ever develop
gout. Therefore, asymptomatic hyperuricemia
does not confer a diagnosis of gout and need
not be treated unless serum uric acid levels
are persistently above 760 μmol/L for men or
600 μmol/L for women. At these levels, there is
an increased risk of renal complications.

- Urate-lowering therapy is typically adjusted to
maintain the serum uric acid below 360 μmol/L.
Lower target urate levels may be required,
depending on the clinical setting.

Common pitfalls

- Uric acid testing is often ordered for patients with
acute monoarthritis. Unfortunately, this will not
be helpful in the diagnosis because of the high
prevalence of asymptomatic hyperuricemia and
the fact that, in 10% of patients with acute gout,
serum uric acid levels are normal. The latter may
be due to increased urinary excretion of uric acid
in the setting of acute inflammation, or possibly
due to sequestration of uric acid into crystal
precipitates in the affected joint.

- The best time to assess the serum uric acid level
is approximately 2 weeks after a gout flare. A
diagnosis of acute gout can only be made with
certainty by joint aspiration to confirm the
presence of urate crystals under polarized light
microscopy.

SYNOVIAL FLUID TESTING

Description

Synovial fluid, obtained by joint aspiration, is
examined visually for viscosity and tested for cell
count and differential, Gram staining, bacteria, and
the presence of crystals under polarized light (see
Table 10.6).

TABLE 10.6. Characteristics of synovial fluid in specific conditions

	Normal	Noninflammatory	Rheumatoid arthritis	Gout or pseudo-gout	Septic arthritis	Hemorrhagic
Colour	Transparent	Transparent	Translucent/opaque	Translucent/opaque	Opaque	Bloody
Viscosity	High	High	Low	Low	Variable	Variable
Gram stain	Negative	Negative	Negative	Negative	Positive	Negative
Bacterial culture	Negative	Negative	Negative	Negative	Positive	Negative
Cell count × 10^6/L	< 200	200–2000	2000–10 000	2000–40 000	> 50 000	200–2000
% PMNs	< 25	< 25	> 50	> 50	> 75	50–75
Crystals	Negative	Negative	Negative	Positive	Negative	Negative

Abbreviation: PMN, polymorphonuclear leukocytes.

Synovial leukocyte count

The synovial leukocyte count is a key piece of information in the investigation of acute inflammatory monoarthritis.

- A WBC count of less than $2000 \times 10^6/L$ indicates a noninflammatory effusion.
- Inflammatory effusions often demonstrate a WBC count of 2000 to $50\,000 \times 10^6/L$.
- Synovial fluid from septic joints usually shows leukocyte counts over $50\,000 \times 10^6/L$, with a predominance of neutrophils. However, these numbers are not absolute, as both lower cell counts and percentage of neutrophils can be seen with septic arthritis, and crystal arthritides can often be associated with leukocyte counts over $50\,000 \times 10^6/L$. However, a leukocyte count higher than $100,000 \times 10^6/L$ and/or percentage of neutrophils more than 90% significantly increases the likelihood of septic arthritis.

Other tests

Other tests of value in specific clinical situations are:

- Gram stain and culture (see chapter 13)
- staining and culture for mycobacteria and fungi
- cytological examination if malignancy is a concern

Examination for crystals

Examination for crystals is done with a polarizing microscope. Microscopy is ideally conducted with a fresh sample of synovial fluid, particularly if looking for calcium pyrophosphate dihydrate (CPPD) crystals. If the clinician lacks equipment or skill to examine the fluid, the laboratory should be alerted to the fact that a fresh specimen must be reviewed as early as possible.

- **Intracellular crystals:** This finding (even in a single cell) is most specific for acute crystal arthritis.

- **Extracellular crystals:** These crystals, especially monosodium urate, can sometimes be seen in synovial fluid between gout attacks.
- **Calcium hydroxyapatite crystals:** These cannot be visualized with routine microscopy.
- **Monosodium urate crystals:** These are associated with gout. They are needle shaped and strongly negatively birefringent (Figure 10.1). These crystals are bright yellow when parallel to the axis of the red compensator of the polarizing microscope. If the position of the crystals, relative to the axis of the compensator, is changed, the crystals will appear bright blue when perpendicular to the axis.
- **CPPD crystals:** These are associated with pseudogout and are weakly positively birefringent and rhomboid shaped (Figure 10.2). These

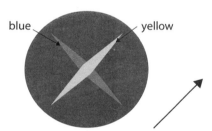

FIGURE 10.1. Monosodium urate: negatively birefringent crystals. Arrow indicates axis of red compensator of polarizing microscope.

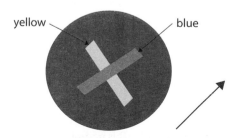

FIGURE 10.2. Calcium pyrophosphate dihydrate (CPPD) positively birefringent crystals. Arrow indicates axis of red compensator of polarizing microscope.

crystals are blue when parallel to the axis of the compensator and yellow when perpendicular.

Common pitfalls

- The most common pitfalls occur when this test is **not** done. Synovial fluid testing must be done to make a diagnosis of infectious or crystal synovitis.

- Synovial fluid chemistry (glucose, lactic dehydrogenase, protein) is of limited value in distinguishing the cause of monoarthritis.

- Because of the tendency of inflammatory and hemorrhagic synovial fluid to clot (thus producing inaccurate cell counts), aspirate samples should be placed into either EDTA or heparinized tubes to facilitate accurate cell count in the laboratory.

- To improve the yield of synovial fluid culture in septic arthritis, synovial aspirates should be inoculated in blood culture vials as well as sterile tubes.

- Sometimes only a small volume of synovial fluid can be obtained. Cell count requires about 1 mL. Culture requires only a few drops for plating, and crystals can be visualized in just a drop or two of fluid (though the laboratory may not accept such a small volume for microscopy). In the setting of acute monoarthritis, the priority is to send fluid for culture and to examine for crystals if limited synovial fluid is available. It is possible for both crystals and infection to be present in the joint.

Further Reading

Agmon-Levin N, Damoiseaux J, Kallenberg C, et al. International recommendations for the assessment of autoantibodies to cellular antigens referred to as antinuclear antibodies. *Ann Rheum Dis.* 2014;73(1):17–23. http://dx.doi.org/10.1136/annrheumdis-2013-203863. Medline:24126457

SELECTION AND INTERPRETATION OF LABORATORY INVESTIGATIONS 207

Finkielman JD, Merkel PA, Schroeder D, et al, and the WGET Research Group. Antiproteinase 3 antineutrophil cytoplasmic antibodies and disease activity in Wegener granulomatosis. *Ann Intern Med.* 2007;147(9):611–9. http://dx.doi.org/10.7326/0003-4819-147-9 -200711060-00005. Medline:17975183

Nielen MM, van Schaardenburg D, Reesink HW, et al. Specific autoantibodies precede the symptoms of rheumatoid arthritis: a study of serial measurements in blood donors. Arthritis Rheum. 2004;50(2):380–6.

Pepys MB, Hirschfield GM. C-reactive protein: a critical update. J Clin Invest. 2003;111(12):1805–12. Erratum in: J Clin Invest. 2003;112(2):299.

Schlesinger N, Norquist JM, Watson DJ. Serum urate during acute gout. J Rheumatol. 2009;36(6):1287–9. Erratum in: J Rheumatol. 2009;36(8):1851.

Sciascia S, Khamashta MA, Bertolaccini ML. New Tests to Detect Antiphospholipid Antibodies: Antiprothrombin (aPT) and Anti-Phosphatidylserine/Prothrombin (aPS/PT) Antibodies. *Curr Rheumatol Rep.* 2014;16(5):415. http://dx.doi.org/10.1007/s11926 -014-0415-x.

Stinton LM, Fritzler MJ. A clinical approach to autoantibody testing in systemic autoimmune rheumatic disorders. *Autoimmun Rev.* 2007;7(1):77–84. http://dx.doi.org/10.1016/j.autrev.2007.08.003. Medline:17967730

Taylor P, Gartemann J, Hsieh, et al. A systematic review of serum biomarkers anti-cyclic citrullinated peptide and rheumatoid factor as tests for rheumatoid arthritis. *Autoimmune Dis [Internet].* 2011 [cited 2013 Nov 15];2011: Article ID 815038 [18 p.] Epub 2011 Sep 11. Available from: http://www.hindawi.com/journals/ ad/2011/815038/

11

Interpretation of Musculoskeletal Imaging

DR. VOLODKO BAKOWSKY
DALHOUSIE UNIVERSITY

Rheumatology is a specialty in which history taking and physical examination are still the most critical elements of patient assessment. However, once this assessment is complete, supporting information from radiologic investigations is often required. These are necessarily guided specifically by the clinical assessment.

Multiple imaging modalities are available. Each of these has its own utility, and set of pros and cons, depending on the anatomic region being studied. The basic principles involved in interpreting these studies are fairly straightforward.

KEY CONCEPTS
1. Imaging studies need to be guided by a thorough history and physical examination.
2. Plain film radiography is usually the first imaging modality used, as it is readily available and inexpensive.
3. A structured approach should be used whenever interpreting joint X-rays. The **ABCDES** framework provides a helpful approach.
4. If additional diagnostic imaging is required, it is important to understand the relative utility, cost, and

availability of other imaging modalities to select the next most appropriate test.

Plain Film Radiography

This section describes standard views for plain film radiographs of specific joints.

- Plain film radiography is almost always the first choice when selecting imaging studies. Plain films offer excellent resolution of bony structures, but are very poor at evaluating soft tissue structures.
- Plain films can differentiate only 4 unique radiodensities—calcium (e.g., bone), water (e.g., muscle, tendon, or joint effusion), fat, and air. Cartilage destruction has to be inferred by narrowing of the joint space.
- Plain films are readily available and low in cost.
- When peripheral joints are evaluated, the patient is exposed to low radiation doses. Spinal and pelvic radiographs require exposure to higher radiation doses and should be selected with greater care, especially in younger patients.
- As plain films of joints are 2-dimensional images of 3-dimensional structures, usually more than 1 profile is required.
  - Before commenting on a study, always look through all the images.
  - For example, joints with contracture may appear to have joint-space narrowing on 1 view, but an alternate view might show that the joint space is actually preserved.
  - This is especially true for X-rays of the fingers and toes.

Imaging

ABBREVIATIONS OF JOINT NOMENCLATURE

CMC: carpometacarpal
DIP: distal interphalangeal
IP: interphalangeal
MCP: metacarpophalangeal
MTP: metatarsophalangeal
PIP: proximal interphalangeal
SI: sacroiliac
TMT: tarsometatarsal

HANDS

- For evaluation of arthritis, often a posterior-anterior (PA) view and ball-catcher's view are adequate. If looking for traumatic changes, a lateral view is also required.
  - The PA view highlights the DIP, PIP, and MCP joints and the carpus (see Figure 11.1).
  - The ball-catcher's view profiles the triquetrum and pisiform and the radial aspect of MCP joints, where early changes can occur in rheumatoid arthritis (RA). In this position, the hands are not held in a fixed position, and therefore reducible subluxations (as in Jaccoud arthropathy, which can occur in lupus) can be visualized (see Figure 11.2).
- Plain X-rays of the hands are often useful in the evaluation of inflammatory arthritis, as changes occur relatively early because the joints are small (a principle that also applies to the feet).
- Bony erosions, and cartilage or joint-space narrowing, tend to develop sooner in the hands and feet compared with large joints such as the knee or hip.
- A standard radiograph of the hands often also allows interpretation of the wrist joints. However,

if the wrist is the predominant area of interest, dedicated wrist views should be obtained.

FEET

- Anteroposterior (AP), oblique, and lateral views are usually obtained.
  - The AP view highlights the IP, MTP, and first and second TMT joints.
  - The oblique view allows visualization of the third to fifth TMT joint.
  - The lateral view profiles the calcaneus, subtalar joint, dorsal aspect of the TMT joints, and insertions of the plantar fascia and Achilles tendons.

SHOULDER

- The 40° posterior oblique view allows profiling of the glenohumeral joint.
- A standard AP view does not profile the glenohumeral joint, but better profiles the acromioclavicular joint.
  - Both visualize the subacromial space.
- "Y" views are usually also obtained routinely:
  - This view is primarily used to look for anterior shoulder dislocation following injury and is less important in rheumatology.
  - The head of the humerus should be centred on the spine of the scapula and proximal humerus, resembling a Mercedes-Benz hood ornament.
  - If this pattern is not present, it can indicate that the shoulder is dislocated.

ELBOW

Standard views include an AP and a lateral view.

HIP

Standard views include an AP of the pelvis and frog-leg lateral positions.

Imaging

KNEE

Standard views include:

- standing AP
  - Remember that considerable joint-space narrowing may be missed by a non-weight-bearing view, as the knee is not compressed by the effect of gravity.

- semiflexed lateral view
  - This view allows evaluation of the patellofemoral joint to some degree, although a dedicated "skyline" view should be obtained for optimal visualization of this joint if desired.

SPINE

- Standard views include an AP and a lateral view.
- Specialized views can include:
  - oblique views of the cervical spine to look for intervertebral foraminal encroachment
  - flexion and extension views of the cervical spine to look for C1–C2 subluxation
  - oblique views of the lumbar spine to look for spondylolysis

SI JOINTS

- These might be seen in a standard AP view of the lumbar spine, but to profile the SI joints specifically, oblique or Hibbs views are often necessary. In this view, the X-ray tube is angled 25° to 30° in a cephalad direction.
- Remember, the key area when looking for sacroiliitis is the inferior one-third of the joint, because this is the synovial portion of the SI joint.
- Pathological changes of the SI joints related to sacroiliitis are usually demonstrated on the iliac side of the joint first, because this side has thinner cartilage.

Approach to Evaluating a Radiograph of a Joint

A systematic and organized approach is helpful when interpreting radiographs. The first step is to learn how to properly describe the abnormalities that you see. The second step is to recognize what patterns of abnormalities occur in different diseases.

A common approach that facilitates X-ray interpretation is **ABCDES** framework:

A: alignment

B: bone

C: cartilage

D: distribution

E: erosions

S: soft tissue

The different radiographic patterns of common types of arthritis according to the **ABCDES** framework are listed in Table 11.1.

ALIGNMENT

- Note the presence of deviation in the alignment of bones, as well as deformities such as joint subluxation and (in its severest form) dislocation.

  - For example, long-standing RA is often associated with deformities such as ulnar deviation of the digits at the MCP joints, as well as swan neck and boutonniere deformities.

- Typically, deviation is described by noting the direction of malalignment of the **distal** segment with respect to the **proximal**.

BONE

Bone changes include an assessment of bone density and new bone formation.

TABLE 11.1. Typical radiographic patterns of common arthritides

Disease	Alignment	Bone	Cartilage	Distribution	Erosions	Soft tissues
Osteoarthritis (OA)	+ Lateral subluxation of digits at IP joints, varus deformity at knee	Density normal Osteophytes, subchondral sclerosis	Nonuniform joint-space narrowing	Involves DIP, PIP, first CMC, AC, hip, knee, first MTP, lumbar and cervical spine Is symmetrical and asymmetrical	Possible central erosions in DIPs and PIPs of hands, none elsewhere	Asymmetrical, if present
Rheumatoid arthritis (RA)	+++ Ulnar deviation at MCP joints, swan neck and boutonniere deformity, valgus deformity at knee (all occur with long-standing disease)	Density normal or reduced	Uniform joint space narrowing	Spares DIP joints and axial skeleton other than C-spine Is symmetrical, usually small joints of hands and feet involved	Marginal erosions	Asymmetrical, if present

(Continued)

TABLE 11.1. (Continued)

Disease	Alignment	Bone	Cartilage	Distribution	Erosions	Soft tissues
Psoriatic arthritis (PsA), spondylarthritis (SpA)	++ As per RA, occasionally arthritis mutilans	Density normal or increased Periosteal new bone formation Fusion distal to wrist and ankles	Uniform joint space narrowing	May be asymmetrical and oligoarticular, "ray pattern," or occasionally RA pattern SI joints and entire spine can be involved, entheses can also be involved	Marginal erosions, occasionally central erosions in small joints of hands	Symmetrical, if present; possible sausage digit
Gout	+ Minimal	Density normal	Preserved joint space until very late	Often has lower extremity predominance	Chronic erosions- elliptical shape with overhanging edge	Asymmetrical, if present
CPPD arthropathy	+ Minimal	Density normal	Uniform or nonuniform loss of cartilage Chondrocalcinosis	Involves MCP joints, shoulder, elbows, wrists and knees Chondrocalcinosis most commonly noted at wrists, knees, and symphysis pubis	No	Symmetrical, if present

Abbreviations: AC, acromioclavicular; CPPD, calcium pyrophosphate dihydrate; C-spine, cervical spine; RA, rheumatoid arthritis; +, abnormalities are present (the more plus signs, the higher the severity).

Imaging

Bone density

- Bone density is a subjective assessment of how radiodense (i.e., how white) the bones look.
- Juxta-articular osteopenia means diminished bone density in the bone surrounding a joint.
  - It can be among the earliest findings in inflammatory arthritis.
  - However, juxta-articular osteopenia can be influenced by the technique of the X-ray study and therefore can lack specificity. Be wary of an X-ray report that mentions juxta-articular osteopenia as the only abnormality.
- In the hand, use the second or third metacarpal to estimate bone density.
  - The sum of the 2 cortices of the shaft of the second or third metacarpal should equal at least one-half its width in a normal digit.
  - If this is not the case, generalized osteopenia is said to be present. This can occur in RA and in osteoporosis.
- Maintenance of normal bone density in the face of changes due to inflammatory arthritis can be a feature of PsA and spondylarthritis (SpA).

New bone formation and calcification

New bone

New bone can manifest in a variety of settings and take a variety of forms:

- **Osteophyte:** This is new bone formed at the margins of affected joints in osteoarthritis (OA).
- **Enthesophyte:** This is new bone formed at sites of tendinous or ligamentous insertion into bone.
  - It can be due to a degenerative process (e.g., a heel spur, or a manifestation of PsA or SpA). The cortical margin of a degenerative enthesophyte is quite clear.

- Entheseal new bone formation secondary to SpA has margins that are somewhat indistinct. It is sometimes accompanied by an erosion in the adjacent bony cortex.

- **New bone beneath articular cartilage:** This is seen in OA. It produces whiter, more radiodense bone (subchondral sclerosis).

- **Periosteal new bone formation in the phalanges**: This can be a sign of PsA or SpA.

- **New bone across joint lines:** This causes fusion or ankylosis.
  - Osteoarthritis can cause fusion of DIP and PIP joints.
  - RA does not cause fusion distal to the wrist or the ankle.
  - PsA and SpA can cause fusion of joints distal to the wrist and ankle and may also cause fusion of the spine and SI joints.

Calcification

Calcification (chondrocalcinosis) is different from new bone formation or ossification.

- The margins of an area of calcification are indistinct, and the radiodensity is lower than that of new bone.

- Calcium pyrophosphate dihydrate (CPPD) deposits may calcify. This may occur in areas of fibrocartilage (e.g., menisci, triangular fibrocartilage of the wrist or symphysis pubis) or in hyaline cartilage.

CARTILAGE

- Joint-space narrowing can be either uniform or nonuniform.
  - Uniform joint space narrowing affects all areas of the joint equally and is typically found in inflammatory arthritis.

- Nonuniform joint-space narrowing is usually a feature of OA (see Figure 11.3). For example, OA of the knee often affects the medial compartment predominantly. In gout, the joint space is often maintained until very late in the disease process.

- Calcification of cartilage (chondrocalcinosis) may be seen in CPPD deposits (see "New Bone Formation and Calcification," above).

DISTRIBUTION

Distribution refers to the number, symmetry, and specific joints affected by the process.

- Rheumatoid arthritis is typically symmetrical.
- SpA affecting the peripheral joints is typically asymmetrical.
- In the hands:
  - RA tends to affect the wrists and multiple MCP and PIP joints.
  - OA affects multiple PIP and DIP joints, as well as the first CMC joint.
  - Psoriatic arthritis and peripheral joint SpA tend to affect digits in a ray pattern: the MCP, the PIP, and even the DIP joints of the same digit.

EROSIONS

Erosions represent a defect in the cortical bone near a joint. They can be marginal or central:

- **Marginal erosions:** These occur in RA, PsA, and SpA. The inflammatory process erodes the bony cortex of the marginal "bare area," where there is no overlying articular cartilage. On a PA view, these types of erosions can look like "mouse ears" (see Figure 11.4).
- In PsA, erosions can cause the bone surrounding the proximal part of the joint to appear whittled

away, while the distal part may show remodelling that creates a cup shape, producing a "pencil-in-a-cup" change (see Figure 11.5).

- **Central erosions:** These are characteristic of the erosive form of OA, and much less frequently PsA and SpA. Central erosions of the DIP and PIP joints in OA can have a "seagull wing" appearance (see Figure 11.3).

- **Erosive OA:** This is a radiographic term that is sometimes confusing.
  - There is no difference between erosive OA and nonerosive OA other than the presence of the central erosions described above.
  - Note that OA does not cause erosive change anywhere other than the hands.

- **Tophi (gout):** Tophi very slowly expand into the bone cortex, allowing the bone to remodel and try to repair itself. This results in "chronic erosions," where an overhanging cortex surrounding the erosion can be visualized (see Figure 11.6).

SOFT TISSUE

- Plain films are not very good at identifying abnormalities in soft tissue. You may, however, be able to see soft tissue swelling surrounding swollen joints.
  - In inflammatory arthritis, this is usually symmetrical around the joint.
  - Asymmetrical soft tissue swelling can occur when there are underlying osteophytes or tophi.
  - Swelling of an entire digit ("sausage digit") is relatively specific for PsA and SpA.

- Calcification of para-articular tendons (e.g., supraspinatus tendon) can also occur and is usually due to hydroxyapatite deposition disease. Calcification of gouty tophi may also occur.

See Figures 11.1 and 11.2 for typical images of normal PA X-rays. See Figures 11.3 to11.7 for images of common arthropathies.

Other Imaging Modalities

ARTHROGRAPHY

- Contrast media can be delivered intra-articularly, under fluoroscopic guidance, into joints such as the shoulder or hip.
- Follow-up imaging done via plain film or CT of the shoulder that notes escape of contrast from the shoulder joint indicates the presence of a full-thickness rotator cuff tear.
- MRI of the hip following gadolinium injection can demonstrate the presence of a labral tear. This technique can also be used to guide therapeutic intra-articular injections.

BONE SCINTIGRAPHY

- Images from bone scintigraphy (also known as a *bone scan*) are typically obtained in 3 phases:
  - **Flow phase:** This is a marker of blood flow to a region, which can be increased for a variety of reasons.
  - **Blood pool:** This can show abnormal radiopharmaceutical uptake due to both bony and soft tissue disease.
  - **Delayed phase:** This is the most important scan for evaluation of bony structures and is obtained several hours after the injection of the radiopharmaceutical. By this time, most uptake that is due to soft tissue problems such as cellulitis should have dissipated.

- A bone scan is a very sensitive technique that can demonstrate areas of early osteomyelitis, stress fractures, avascular necrosis, and metastatic disease much earlier than plain films. It can also identify diseased joints, because the para-articular bone often lights up on the scan.
- The resolution of these images has historically not been very good. However, bone scans are now often done in association with a localizing CT; the amount of uptake of radiopharmaceutical is superimposed on the CT slices to provide much greater resolution. The localizing CT is not as good as a dedicated CT, but it is still often good enough to detect erosive disease.
- Bone scans can either be regional (e.g., of the lower extremity) if one is looking for a stress fracture, or full body, depending on the indication.

CT SCANS

- CT scans provide much better soft tissue contrast than plain films. They can demonstrate bony changes earlier than plain film in osteomyelitis or avascular necrosis.
- They are also of great help in evaluating the cross-sectional anatomy of structures that are too complex to be well visualized with plain film (e.g., hindfoot, SI joints, and sternoclavicular joints).
- They are often more readily available than MRI. A CT scan is frequently the initial imaging study of choice for patients with suspected lumbosacral nerve root impingement, due to its availability, even though it is slightly inferior to MRI.
- The amount of radiation delivered by a CT scan is a concern.
  - This is particularly important in younger and female patients.

Imaging

- For this reason, CT scans are rarely, if ever, used in pediatric patients.

- CT scans of joints, unlike body scans, rarely require the administration of IV contrast and therefore tend to be safer in patients with renal insufficiency (IV contrast is nephrotoxic).

- A new technique—dual energy CT—is available at some centres. This technique allows for identification of deposits of uric acid and can facilitate a diagnosis of gout.

MAGNETIC RESONANCE IMAGING

MRI scanning has become an essential imaging technique for a variety of musculoskeletal problems. It derives structural information from the density of protons that differ in various types of tissue.

The mechanism of magnetic resonance imaging

About 10% of the body is composed of the element hydrogen. Some hydrogen exists in its ionized form (loses its electron)—in other words, as protons. A proton has a magnetic charge and spin; however, each proton is slightly different, because there is no organized pattern. MRIs deliver a strong external magnetic charge that lines up the protons in the body and makes them all spin in the same direction. Tissues exhibit contrast by giving off signals that differ according to how quickly their protons return to a normal state.

A full understanding of MRI principles is beyond the scope of this chapter, but some basics include:

- Different MRI sequences can be chosen by the radiologist to highlight certain specific pathological features. Different sequences are produced by adjusting the specifics of the excitation and relaxation of the protons.

TABLE 11.2. Characteristic tissue signals on MRI

MRI sequence	Cortical bone	Muscle	Ligament and tendon	Water, edema, and inflammation	Bone marrow and fat
T1	Dark	Intermediate	Dark	Dark	Bright
T2	Dark	Intermediate	Dark	Bright	Intermediate

- Two sequences that are almost always included in a standard MRI study are T1-weighted and T2-weighted images. Table 11.2 outlines characteristic signals of various tissues.
- Pathological processes (infiltrative disease, infection, and bone marrow edema) have a low signal on a T1 study.
- Synovial fluid, edema, and cysts are bright on T2 images.
- There are other sequences known as "fat suppressed" techniques, such as short tau inversion recovery (STIR), which often demonstrate edema better than in T2 images by reducing the signal returned from fatty tissue such as bone marrow.

Indications for MRI

- Indications for MRI are extensive, and MRI may be the best imaging modality available in some cases.
  - MRI is the investigation of choice for imaging soft tissue masses; internal derangement of the knee; avascular necrosis, cervical spine cord or nerve root disease; lumbosacral spine nerve root disease; and early osteomyelitis, to name a few.
  - In rheumatology, MRI is the study of choice to detect early, nonradiographic sacroiliitis and spondylitis in the diagnosis of SpA (see chapter 8).
  - MRI can also detect rotator cuff tears, synovitis, and tenosynovitis.

Imaging

- It can be performed with intra-articular or IV gadolinium contrast enhancement. The former technique can help diagnose subtle abnormalities such as labral tears of the hip. The latter technique can identify synovial proliferation from inflammatory arthritis.

- Previously, MRI imaging with contrast was preferred for patients with renal insufficiency, as CT contrast is nephrotoxic. However, a disease that mimics scleroderma, nephrogenic systemic fibrosis, has been described in patients with chronic kidney disease who receive IV gadolinium, and therefore gadolinium enhancement is now avoided in these patients.

- MRI scanning is, unfortunately, a time-consuming process. What takes a few seconds of imaging time on CT may take 15 to 30 minutes with MRI. This can make this valuable imaging modality difficult to access.

- During imaging, patients have to remain very still in a small space and claustrophobic patients may have difficulty tolerating the study.

- Contraindications to MRI scans include imbedded metal fragments (especially ocular, for example, in metal workers) and implanted pacemakers.
  - Newer implanted technological devices are increasingly being made "MRI friendly."
  - It is important to check the composition of any implanted devices, as well as checking with the MRI technicians, before denying a patient a needed MRI.

- MRI does not deliver any radiation to patients, and therefore may be preferentially selected in children, younger patients, and women of childbearing age.

POSITRON EMISSION TOMOGRAPHY SCANS

Positron emission tomography (PET) is a relatively new imaging technology. It combines the injection of a radiotracer, ^{18}F-fluorodeoxyglucose (FDG), with a CT-like detector. The radioactive glucose tracer becomes concentrated in areas of increased glucose metabolism (such as sites of malignancy, infection, and other inflammatory disorders) and localization is facilitated by an array of detectors that receive signals emitted by the radiotracer. A computer reassembles the signals into images that reveal differences in metabolic activity between healthy and diseased tissue.

- PET is currently only available in larger urban centres.
- PET scans are primarily available for the workup and monitoring of patients with malignancies.
- In rheumatology, these studies are used in some centres for the assessment of large vessel vasculitis.
- A PET scan will show inflamed joints, but it is not currently used for that purpose.

ULTRASOUND

Ultrasound uses high-frequency sound waves and the echo they return to obtain an image of tissue. The sound waves travel into tissue and, where there is a junction between 2 types of tissue, some of the sound waves bounce back. Other waves continue into the tissue until the next interface. An ultrasound probe detects the waves that bounce back. All of the sound waves that bounce back are collected to form an image.

- Ultrasound is increasingly being used for musculoskeletal imaging.
  - It can be used to evaluate the integrity of the rotator cuff and Achilles tendons.

- It can be valuable in detecting synovitis in difficult-to-examine joints such as the MTP joints.

• As with MRI, ultrasound involves no radiation exposure.

• **Bedside ultrasonography** is increasingly being practiced by clinical rheumatologists in a targeted fashion, as an adjunct to physical examination. It may well become a routinely used tool.

- These techniques can be especially helpful in patients with extensively damaged joints when there is a question about residual inflammatory activity, and in patients with a technically difficult examination, such as obese patients.
- Doppler ultrasound can measure blood flow to joints; increased blood flow correlates with joint inflammation.
- The presence of synovitis and erosion-like changes can be detected with ultrasound before detection by physical examination and X-ray.
- The use of bedside ultrasonography enhances the clinician's ability to make an early diagnosis of inflammatory arthritis and initiate appropriate therapy.

Examples of Hand Radiographs in Various Arthropathies

The hand radiographs that follow (Figures 11.1 to 11.7) provide examples of characteristic findings in arthropathies.

An understanding of the radiographic features of different arthropathies on plain film radiography is an essential skill for assessing patients with arthritis. A standardized approach can be helpful in classifying radiographic findings. After that, it is a matter of pattern recognition to identify the disease that best matches the radiograph.

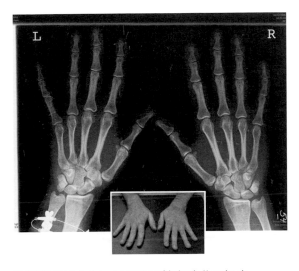

FIGURE 11.1. Posterior-anterior X-ray of the hands. Normal study. Inset: Correct positioning of hands for X-ray.

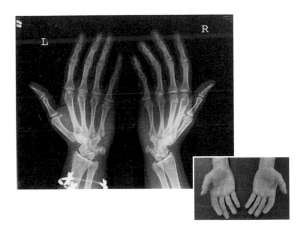

FIGURE 11.2. Ball-catcher's view of the hands. Inset: Correct positioning of the hands for X-ray.

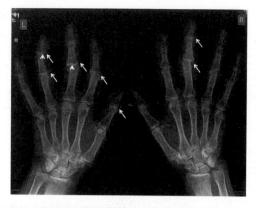

FIGURE 11.3. Osteoarthritis. Alignment findings include ulnar deviation of the bilateral third and left second finger middle phalanges at the PIP joint, as well as flexion deformity of the left fourth finger at the DIP joint. Bone density is normal. Osteophytes are present at the right third finger PIP and DIP and left thumb IP, PIP #2-4, and the fourth finger DIP joints (arrows). Nonuniform joint-space narrowing is evident in most of these same joints. The joints involved are predominantly the PIP and DIP joints. Central erosions are present in the left fourth finger DIP and the left third PIP joints (arrowheads). These have the appearance of "seagull wings." There is increased soft tissue density surrounding the right third PIP and left second PIP joints.

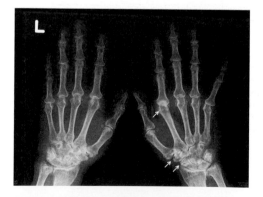

FIGURE 11.4. Rheumatoid arthritis. Alignment findings include ulnar deviation of the right fifth finger at the MCP joint, radial deviation of the left wrist, and volar subluxation of the right second MCP joint. Both generalized osteopenia and para-articular osteopenia are present, most notably at the right wrist and the left MCP joints. Bilateral pan-carpal joint-space narrowing is present, along with uniform joint-space narrowing at the MCPs bilaterally. The joints involved are primarily the wrists and MCPs. Marginal erosions are best visualized in the right second MCP joint and right carpus (arrows). There are no soft tissue abnormalities in this example.

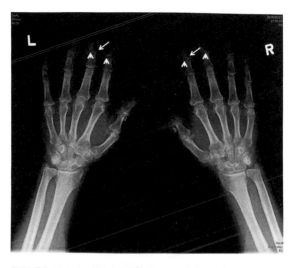

FIGURE 11.5. Psoriatic arthritis. Alignment findings include marked radial subluxation of the right thumb distal phalanx, as well as ulnar subluxation of the left third finger distal phalanx. Mild flexion deformity is present in the right second and third DIP joints. Bone density is preserved. There is no periosteal bone formation as can sometimes be seen in psoriatic arthritis. Joint-space narrowing occurs in the right second finger and left third finger DIP joints (arrows). The joints involved are primarily the DIP joints of both hands and the IP joint of the left thumb. Central erosions are present at the DIP joints of the right and left second and third fingers (arrowheads). These destructive erosions give the appearance of joint widening in the right third finger and left second finger DIP joints. The left second DIP has the early appearance of "pencil in a cup" due to remodelling of the proximal aspect of the distal phalanx such that it looks cup shaped. There is increased soft tissue density surrounding both second finger DIP joints, as well as subtle joint-space narrowing of the second and third MCP of the right hand. (The calcification just proximal to the IP joint of the left thumb is an incidental finding.)

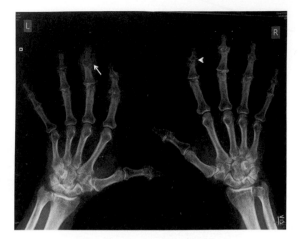

FIGURE 11.6. Gout. Alignment findings include mild ulnar deviation of the distal phalanx of both second digits at the DIP joint and radial deviation of the left third finger distal phalanx. Bone density is preserved. Joint-space narrowing and osteophyte formation involving multiple DIP joints are present due to concomitant osteoarthritis. The joints to focus on in this image, however, are the left third finger and right second finger DIP joints. The joint space of the left third finger DIP has been completely destroyed by a very large erosion (arrow). Multiple erosions can be seen in the right second finger DIP, including 1 on the ulnar aspect of the joint that appears to have an overhanging cortical edge (arrowhead)—a "chronic erosion" because it has developed slowly enough that the bone has had time to try to repair itself. Increased soft tissue density surrounds the left third finger DIP, second PIP joints, and right second DIP joint. The soft tissue density overlying the left third finger DIP joint has a "lumpy and bumpy" appearance compatible with tophaceous deposition. One characteristic feature of gout not demonstrated here is the preservation of joint space until very late in the disease.

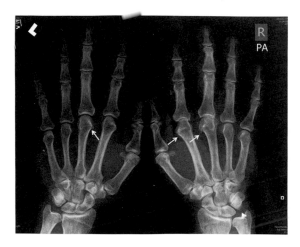

FIGURE 11.7. Calcium pyrophosphate dihydrate (CPPD) arthritis.
The alignment is normal. Bone density is preserved. "Hook like" osteophytes are present at the right second and third finger and left third finger MCP joints (arrows). There is uniform joint-space narrowing at these joints as well, most notably at the right third finger MCP joint. There is no calcification of hyaline cartilage. No erosions are present. Soft tissues are normal. There is no calcification of the triangular fibrocartilage (arrows), which is sometimes seen with CPPD deposition. These changes are predominantly those of osteoarthritis (OA); however, primary OA does not occur to this degree in the MCP joints. Thus, secondary causes of OA, such as CPPD deposition, should be considered.

Further Reading

Brower AC, Flemming DJ. Arthritis in black and white. 3rd ed. Philadelphia: Saunders; 2012.

Hochberg MC, Silman AJ, Smolen JS, et al, editors. Rheumatology. 6th ed. Maryland Heights (MO): Mosby; 2014.

Manaster BJ, May DA, Disler DG. Musculoskeletal imaging: the requisites. 4th ed. Philadelphia: Saunders; 2013.

For further information regarding bedside ultrasonography:

Canadian Rheumatology Ultrasound Society [Internet]. c2010 CRUS-SURC [cited 2014 Sep 6]. Available from: http://crus-surc.ca/

SECTION 3: APPROACH TO THERAPEUTICS

12

Pharmacologic Therapy

DR. LORI ALBERT
UNIVERSITY OF TORONTO

KEY CONCEPTS

1. Some therapeutic agents, such as nonsteroidal anti-inflammatory drugs (NSAIDs), can be used to manage mild and nonspecific symptoms. However, therapy with glucocorticoids (GCs) and other immunosuppressive agents should only be undertaken after every effort has been made to clarify the diagnosis.

2. Although it is advisable to avoid polypharmacy, combinations of drugs are often required in treating rheumatic diseases.

3. Most drugs used to manage rheumatic diseases have potentially serious side effects, and regular monitoring of clinical status and blood work is required to manage this risk. Some toxicity can also be avoided by preemptive treatment with other agents (e.g., prevention of steroid-induced osteoporosis with a bisphosphonate).

4. It is essential that patients be educated about their condition and the rationale for the therapeutic plan to encourage adherence. Patients should be counselled carefully on the potential side effects and appropriate monitoring of drugs. Drug choices may need to be modified according to patient acceptance and willingness to adhere to monitoring regimens.

Note: This section provides an overview to the use of:

- nonsteroidal anti-inflammatory drugs (NSAIDs)
- glucocorticoids (GCs)
- disease-modifying antirheumatic drugs (DMARDs): conventional and biologic

Further reading or consultation with a rheumatologist is required for optimal use of these agents.

Nonsteroidal Anti-inflammatory Drugs (NSAIDs)

Therapeutics

USES

- In rheumatology, NSAIDs are used for their analgesic and mild anti-inflammatory properties.
- NSAIDs are useful for symptomatic relief, but do not have disease-modifying properties for chronic inflammatory conditions. In acute inflammatory conditions (e.g., bursitis, acute crystal arthritis), they alone may be sufficient therapy.
- There are several classes of these drugs, which are based on their structure. It has been found empirically that if a drug from 1 class is ineffective, a different NSAID may be tried with better effect.
- The primary site of NSAID action is the cyclooxygenase enzyme (COX) that converts arachidonic acid into prostaglandins, which play an important role in mediating inflammation and pain. Two forms of this enzyme have been described, COX-1 and COX-2:
  - **COX-1** is normally present in high concentrations in platelets, vascular endothelial cells, stomach, and kidney-collecting tubules. It is responsible for the production of prostaglandins that are essential for maintenance of normal endocrine

and renal function, gastric mucosal integrity, and hemostasis.

- **COX-2** is now known to be expressed in many tissues, but is upregulated by inflammatory stimuli. It is responsible for the production of inflammatory prostaglandins. NSAIDs do not suppress leukotriene synthesis by lipoxygenase pathways.

- Most NSAIDs currently available in North America are nonselective and inhibit both COX-1 and COX-2.
  - A second class of NSAIDs (coxibs) was developed to selectively inhibit COX-2 in an effort to reduce side effects, particularly GI side effects, resulting from inhibition of COX-1.
  - Only 1 of these drugs is currently available: others that were developed were associated with cardiovascular and cerebrovascular toxicity and were removed from the market.

SIDE EFFECTS

- NSAIDs are tolerated well by most individuals using them for short duration; overall risk of serious complications is low for short-term use in healthy individuals.
  - With prolonged treatment, or in the presence of comorbidities, the risks may be higher.
  - For an individual patient, the risk-benefit ratio must be considered when prescribing these agents.
  - Consider whether an alternative agent, such as acetaminophen, will provide the therapeutic outcome that is desired.

- Given the frequent use of these agents, a more extensive list of side effects is reviewed here than for other agents, but the discussion that follows is not exhaustive.

Gastrointestinal side effects

- If patients develop dyspepsia, gastroesophageal reflux disease, or nausea:
  - Patients may tolerate a different NSAID.
  - Patients can be coprescribed an H2-blocker, proton pump inhibitor, or misoprostol.

- Serious side effects include peptic ulcer disease and its complications. This may be **asymptomatic**, especially if in the more distal segments.

- Gastroduodenal endoscopic erosions or ulcers develop in 20% to 40% of patients within 3 months of starting therapy.

- Patients can present with a slow, subclinical bleed (anemia, fatigue) or with acute hemorrhage.

- Patients may present with ulcer complications such as perforation and stricture.

- The distal small bowel and colon are also susceptible to these complications, including the formation of strictures, called diaphragms, which can cause bowel obstruction.

Risk factors

- Identified risk factors for clinical gastroduodenal events include: prior history of an upper GI event (ulcers and complications); age 60 or more years; multiple NSAID use (including ASA); high-dose NSAID use; prolonged NSAID use; concomitant anticoagulant use; low-dose ASA use; concomitant GC use; and probably concomitant use of bisphosphonates and selective serotonin reuptake inhibitors (SSRIs).

- Use of enteric-coated or sustained-release formulations is likely a risk factor for distal segment disease.

- Compared with nonselective NSAIDs, coxibs may be associated with lower risk of gastroduodenal

Therapeutics

events, but can still cause GI intolerance in older patients. Coxibs may not be protective against GI events in distal segments of the bowel.

- Treatment of NSAID-induced injuries is discontinuation of the NSAID.
- To reduce the risk of NSAID-induced injury, it is recommended that patients be prescribed a proton pump inhibitor (or misoprostol) if taking an NSAID, even in combination with a coxib, in patients that are at higher risk. NSAIDs should be avoided in those with risk factors for toxicity, particularly the elderly and those on anticoagulants.

Renal and circulatory side effects

Prostaglandins act locally in the kidney to maintain homeostasis by regulating sodium and water reabsorption, particularly in the thick ascending loop of Henle and the collecting duct. Through prostaglandin inhibition, NSAIDs increase sodium and water retention by increasing the tubular reabsorption of sodium.

All NSAIDs and coxibs can produce toxicity from possible:

- electrolyte and fluid retention
  - This can lead to congestive heart failure or worsening of congestive heart failure.
  - Sodium retention can lead to edema.
  - Potassium retention can lead to hyperkalemia.
- hypertension (other mechanisms as well)
  - Patients with hypertension or borderline hypertension are at higher risk of this side effect.
  - Elderly patients are at higher risk.
  - This side effect is less common in normotensive healthy individuals, but BP should be monitored in all chronic NSAID users.

- acute kidney injury and chronic kidney disease
  - Patients receiving concomitant angiotensin-converting enzyme inhibitors, angiotensin receptor blockers and diuretics, and aminoglycosides have a higher risk of acute kidney injury.
- acute papillary necrosis
- acute tubulointerstitial nephritis

Hepatic side effects
- Elevations in hepatic transaminases are commonly associated with NSAIDs. Liver failure is rare.
- Elevations may be disease specific: there is evidence for increased risk of hepatotoxic reactions in patients with systemic lupus erythematosus (SLE).

Cardiovascular side effects
- The mechanism of risk is multifactorial. Cardiovascular side effects may be due, in part, to degree of COX-2 selectivity associated with reduced prostaglandin I_2 production and reduced inhibition of platelet thromboxane A_2.
- Risk of major cardiovascular events such as myocardial infarction, stroke, atrial fibrillation, and cardiovascular death is increased by all NSAIDs (nonselective and coxibs), especially at high doses (mainly an issue with chronic use rather than short-term use).
- Naproxen does not appear to have the same risks as other NSAIDs at high doses (the risk is higher with low doses). Diclofenac may have the highest risk: maximum daily dose should not exceed 100 mg.
- NSAIDs carry a risk of heart failure, particularly

Therapeutics

in the setting of underlying cardiovascular disease.

- They carry a risk of hypertension, particularly in those with preexisting hypertension.

Hematologic side effects

- Antiplatelet effect is due to inhibition of COX-1.

- Avoid NSAIDs in patients with thrombocytopenia or preexisting platelet defects (consider a coxib).

- NSAIDs should be held at least 3 days before surgery (for ASA, 1 week is required to produce new platelets, since COX in platelets is irreversibly inhibited by ASA).

- NSAIDs cannot be assumed to replace ASA for cardiovascular protection; thus, low-dose ASA may need to be continued, with attendant increased GI risk. In addition, ibuprofen (and possibly other NSAIDs) may reduce effectiveness of ASA for cardiovascular protection.

- Neutropenia rarely occurs.

Central nervous system side effects

- Aseptic meningitis is more prevalent in patients with SLE.

- Psychosis and cognitive impairment are more prevalent in older patients, especially with indomethacin use (many patients note headaches or unusual feelings of depersonalization).

Other side effects

- These can include bronchospasm, skin rashes, and anaphylaxis.

- Note that the risks of NSAID in pregnancy are not clear (ASA is sometimes used in the setting of antiphospholipid antibody syndrome). NSAIDs should not be used after 30 weeks of gestation due to risk of premature closure of ductus arteriosus.

Topical NSAIDs

- Two preparations of topical diclofenac are currently available.
- Clinical trials suggest that efficacy is similar to oral NSAIDs with fewer GI effects.
- The cardiovascular and renal safety profiles have not been established.
- The use of topical NSAIDs would be preferable to oral NSAIDs in older patients with osteoarthritis.

Glucocorticoids

USES

These drugs are an important part of the armamentarium of the rheumatologist. There are 2 main indications for GCs:

- suppression of the inflammatory cascade
- modification of the immune response

FORMULATIONS USED

The following are equivalent: prednisone 5 mg, methylprednisolone (Solu-Medrol) 4 mg, and hydrocortisone (Solu-Cortef) 20 mg.

GCs bind to receptors in the cytoplasm and produce their effects by:

- nongenomic activation of anti-inflammatory proteins
- DNA-dependent regulation of anti-inflammatory proteins (GC/receptor complex binds to GC-responsive elements of genome)
- protein interference mechanisms (GC/receptor complex binds to nuclear-factor- κβ-responsive

elements to prevent transcription of pro-inflammatory cytokines)

There are also nonspecific, nongenomic membrane effects at high doses. At high concentrations, GCs are able to intercalate into cellular membranes and change their properties. This may be the mechanism behind the rapid benefits of pulse Solu-Medrol therapy, or intra-articular injections of GCs.

High-dose therapy
- High-dose therapy starts at 40 mg/d prednisone and goes up to 1 mg/kg/d.
- Typical scenarios for high-dose therapy include:
  - systemic vasculitis with organ involvement (e.g., granulomatosis with polyangiitis, polyarteritis nodosa, or temporal arteritis)
  - polymyositis or dermatomyositis
  - SLE flare involving kidney, CNS, mononeuritis multiplex, transverse myelitis, severe thrombocytopenia, lung, or other significant organ involvement

- High-dose therapy is usually continued for a month before proceeding with a taper.
- Pulse therapy (e.g., methylprednisolone 1 g IV once daily for 3 days) is a unique way of giving very high doses of GCs over a short period, with the intention of rapidly suppressing an acute inflammatory process.
  - It may be considered when the disease is producing life-threatening or organ-threatening complications.
  - After the "pulse," high-dose therapy is resumed.
  - Pulse therapy is associated with a significantly higher risk of side effects.
  - It has been suggested that in treating severe lupus, lower doses (250 mg or 500 mg) may be adequate.

Low- or moderate-dose therapy

- Low-dose corticosteroid therapy is usually defined as less than 15 mg prednisone. A moderate dose is 15–40 mg.

- Low- and moderate-dose therapy is used for less severe disease or in other conditions where a lesser degree of immune modulation is required.

- Settings in which moderate dosing would be considered include SLE with less significant organ involvement, or vasculitis with less significant organ involvement and/or good prognostic features (see chapter 5).

- Settings in which low-dose GCs would be considered include polymyalgia rheumatica, or as adjunctive therapy in severe rheumatoid arthritis while waiting for other DMARDs to work.

TAPERING GCs

- Once disease control has been established, high prednisone doses should be tapered.

- While there are various tapering protocols for specific diseases, a few general principles are usually followed.

  - In patients receiving doses of prednisone greater than 30 mg/d, the dose can be tapered relatively rapidly at rates of 5–10 mg/wk.
  - When the dose is below 20 mg/d, the dose should be tapered by 2.5–5 mg every 2 to 4 weeks.
  - When patients are taking 10 mg or less, a common practice is to taper prednisone in decrements of 1–2.5 mg each month.

- Tapering requires attention to disease activity; therefore, measures of disease activity in the individual must be established at the outset of treatment and a decision made as to what

Therapeutics

will constitute a flare versus maintenance of disease control. Measures of activity may be **established indices** (e.g., Disease Activity Score in rheumatoid arthritis, Systemic Lupus Erythematosus Disease Activity Index in lupus); **laboratory indices** relevant to organ involvement (e.g., creatinine or proteinuria in lupus nephritis); or **specific disease markers** that are responsive to treatment (e.g., serum complement levels in a particular lupus patient).

- **Note**: Some patients experience a steroid withdrawal phenomenon, with aching, stiffness, and malaise during the first 1 or 2 weeks of transition to a lower dose of prednisone.

- When withdrawing long-term GC therapy, an adrenocorticotropic hormone (ACTH) stimulation test may be appropriate but is not mandatory. Adrenal insufficiency may develop upon GC discontinuation and the risk persists for up to 1 year, especially if the patient is stressed by infection or surgery.

PERIOPERATIVE GC COVERAGE

Indications

Supplemental GC coverage should be considered for any patient who has received corticosteroids for more than a few weeks in the previous year.

- Generally, supplemental steroids are administered to all patients who have been taking GCs who are seriously ill or undergoing major surgery.

- It is possible to test the integrity of the hypothalamic-pituitary-adrenal axis using an ACTH stimulation test. However, this test is difficult to interpret in critically ill patients and a formal test is usually unnecessary in this setting.

Dose

The dose required for perioperative GC coverage is not high. For most moderately severe acute illnesses, continuation of the current dose of GC is adequate, but supplementation may be reasonable.

- Physiological cortisol secretion in response to major surgery is approximately 75–150 mg/d; return to baseline occurs 24 to 48 hours after surgery.
- Traditional perioperative protocols provide more GC than is needed, but have become established regimens.
  - **Major surgery:** A reasonable protocol is hydrocortisone 100 mg IV with anesthetic induction and every 8 hours thereafter for up to 72 hours.
  - **Moderate surgery or major febrile illness:** Patients may take their usual dose of oral prednisone on the day of surgery followed by 50–75 mg of hydrocortisone IV immediately preoperatively and every 8 hours thereafter for 48 to 72 hours.
  - **Minor procedures or mild febrile illness:** Patients may take their usual dose of oral prednisone on the day of surgery and 25 mg of hydrocortisone IV immediately preoperatively; patients can return to their usual prednisone dose on the second postoperative day. Other protocols suggest even shorter duration of therapy.
- Mineralocorticoid supplementation is usually not required in patients on long-term GC therapy. Longer acting methylprednisolone can be used for supplementation perioperatively.
- Patients undergoing superficial procedures of less than 1 hour (e.g., skin biopsy, dental work) require

only their normal daily dose of replacement therapy and not a supplemental dose.

ADVERSE EFFECTS

Adverse effects of GCs are largely related to dose and duration of therapy. Some adverse effects include:

- glucose intolerance
- edema and hypertension
- osteoporosis (doses greater than 5–7.5 mg/d) (50% of patients will lose bone mass)
- weight gain and obesity
- skin manifestations (easy bruising, striae, impaired wound healing)
- cataract formation (even with 5mg/d for prolonged periods)
- avascular necrosis
- infection (doses greater than 0.3 mg/kg)
- hirsutism
- abnormal menstruation
- mood swings, agitation, sleeplessness, and/or psychosis (rare)
- muscle weakness (doses greater than 10–20 mg/d)
- peptic ulcer disease (when combined with NSAIDs)

Most adverse effects are not preventable, but do require close monitoring. Institution of therapy to prevent GC-induced osteoporosis should be considered (see chapter 9).

INTRA-ARTICULAR STEROIDS

The judicious use of this form of steroid therapy can provide excellent relief of inflammatory arthritis in the setting of noninfectious mono- or polyarthritis. This may also allow for minimization of systemic GCs for inflammatory arthritis.

Indications

Indications include:

- monoarthritis (after joint infection is ruled out)
- disproportionate inflammation of 1 or 2 joints in a patient with polyarthritis (after infection is ruled out)
- tendon sheath inflammation
- bursitis or tendinitis refractory to NSAIDs

Intra-articular injection should only be undertaken if the operator is confident about how to enter the joint or tendon sheath (see chapter 19). Ideally, fluid should be withdrawn from the joint before injection to ensure proper needle placement. If resistance is met during injection, the needle should be withdrawn and repositioned.

Complications of steroid injection
Infection:
Several complications can arise from steroid injection, and many are related to skill and technique. Complications include:

- This is rare, but aseptic technique must be ensured.
- Avoid infected skin lesions, or open wounds around the joint.
- Prosthetic joints should not be injected.

Hypopigmentation of local skin

Subcutaneous tissue atrophy

Hemarthrosis: This is rare, except in patients with coagulopathy.

Tendon rupture: This may occur if steroid is injected directly into tendon rather than the joint.

Steroid-crystal-induced synovitis ("postinjection flare"):

- It may be avoided by agitating the steroid solution before injection.

- Patients should be warned that this can occur but is not serious and can be managed conservatively with ice application and analgesics.

Cartilage damage or tendon weakening:
- This is a theoretical risk if injections are given more frequently than every 3 to 4 months.
- If repeat injections are required, consider whether systemic therapy is appropriate or needs adjustment.
- There is some suppression of cortisol levels for up to 7 days postinjection, but this is rarely clinically relevant.
- Transient elevation of blood glucose may occur in patients with diabetes.

Other considerations

Consider the following factors in decisions about intra-articular steroids:

- patient acceptance of injection
- patient use of anticoagulants
- preexisting joint instability
- lack of response to previous injections
- accessibility of joint
- presence of infection locally or systemically

Preparations

Note that the availability of preparations may vary from province to province.

Dexamethasone sodium phosphate (Decadron): This has fast onset and shorter duration of action.

Methylprednisolone acetate (Depo-Medrol): This has intermediate onset and duration of action up to 3 to 4 months or longer.

Triamcinolone acetonide (Kenalog) or triamcinolone hexacetonide (Aristospan): This has slower onset and prolonged duration of action.

Dosing depends on the preparation used and joint size (see Tables 12.1a and 12.1b).

TABLE 12.1a. Typical dosing for intra-articular injection of methylprednisolone acetate (Depo-Medrol)

Area	Dose
Finger joint (MCP, PIP)	10 mg
Wrist	20 mg
Elbow	20–40 mg
Shoulder	40 mg
Hip	80–120 mg
Knee	40–80 mg
Ankle	40 mg

TABLE 12.1b. Typical dosing for intra-articular injection of triamcinolone preparations

Preparation	Large joint	Small joint
Triamcinolone hexacetonide (Aristospan)	10–20 mg	2–6 mg
Triamcinolone acetonide (Kenalog)	40 mg (knee, shoulder)	10 mg
	30 mg (wrist, elbow, ankle)	

Anesthetic preparations can be safely mixed with corticosteroid preparations, but the total volume must be kept in mind—overdistending the joint should be avoided.

Disease-Modifying Antirheumatic Drugs (DMARDs)

- DMARDs slow the progress or damage induced by a particular disease. The term *DMARD* primarily refers to drugs used to treat rheumatoid arthritis—these drugs do more than treat symptoms: they have been shown to prevent or slow erosive radiographic change.
- In practice, for nonrheumatoid arthritis diseases, many of these same drugs are used as "steroid sparing" agents to modify the immune

response and allow the dose of prednisone to be substantially tapered or discontinued.

- The development of therapy with conventional DMARDs or steroid-sparing agents has been largely empirical.

- The development of "targeted" therapeutics in immune-mediated diseases is the result of improved understanding of inflammatory pathways and recognition of specific molecular targets.

  - **Biologic response modifiers or "biologics"** are primarily monoclonal antibodies used for therapeutic purposes. These are large proteins that require IV or subcutaneous administration. Antibodies or antibody-like proteins that target inflammatory cytokines or immune cell surface receptors have been developed. Examples of targets include tumour necrosis factor α (TNF-α), interleukin 6 (IL-6), costimulatory molecules, and others.

  - **"Small molecule inhibitors"** target intracellular kinases, which are important for signal transmission in cells of the immune system. Other intracellular targets are being explored. These therapies are typically administered orally.

MOST COMMONLY USED DMARDs

Details of these drugs are beyond the scope of this book. Table 12.2 presents a summary for quick reference.

For rheumatoid arthritis and other inflammatory arthritides

- hydroxychloroquine (Plaquenil)
- sulfasalazine (Salazopyrin)
- methotrexate

TABLE 12.2. Commonly used DMARDs and immunosuppressives: side effects and monitoring

Drug	Common uses	Side effects	Monitoring
Plaquenil	Early RA; SLE; rash in DM	Ocular toxicity	Yearly field tests with or without OCT with ophthalmologist
Sulfasalazine	RA, PsA, and other peripheral SpA	GI, rash, bone marrow suppression, liver (rare)	Monthly blood work for CBC, liver enzymes
Methotrexate*	RA; PsA; SLE with arthritis (steroid sparing); vasculitis (some); myositis	Elevated liver enzymes, bone marrow suppression, pneumonitis (rare)	Monthly blood work for CBC, AST, ALT, creatinine
Leflunomide	RA; PsA; arthritis in SLE (sometimes used)	Elevated liver enzymes, bone marrow suppression, GI toxicity	Monthly blood work for CBC, AST, ALT
Gold sodium thiomalate	RA (uncommonly used)	Rash, cytopenias, membranous nephritis	Monthly CBC, liver enzymes, creatinine, urinalysis
Azathioprine	SLE (steroid sparing), other collagen vascular diseases	Bone marrow suppression, infection, idiosyncratic hepatitis, interstitial nephritis (rare)	Monthly blood work for CBC, liver enzymes
Cyclophosphamide	Serious manifestations of SLE, vasculitis	Infection; cytopenias; hemorrhagic cystitis; infertility; bladder cancer (long-term risk)	Regular CBC, urinalysis, cytology every 3–6 months
Mycophenolate mofetil, mycophenolic acid	SLE, especially lupus nephritis	Infection, cytopenias, GI intolerance, elevated liver enzymes	Regular CBC, liver enzymes
Cyclosporine	Occasionally: SLE, RA, PsA, inflammatory myositis, and some other settings	Nephrotoxicity, hypertension, neurotoxicity, infection, malignancy, hyperuricemia, metabolic abnormalities	Regular monitoring of BP, creatinine, BUN, liver enzymes, glucose, magnesium, potassium Cyclosporine levels (can be followed early in therapy)

Abbreviations: DM, dermatomyositis; OCT, optical coherence tomography; PsA, psoriatic arthritis; RA, rheumatoid arthritis; SLE, systemic lupus erythematosus; SpA, spondylarthritis.

*Use with folic acid.

Therapeutics

- leflunomide (Arava)
- gold sodium thiomalate (Myochrysine)

For systemic lupus erythematosus
- hydroxychloroquine
- azathioprine (Imuran)
- mycophenolate mofetil (Cellcept) or mycophenolic acid (Myfortic)
- cyclophosphamide (Cytoxan) (preferably avoided except for severe disease manifestations)
- cyclosporine (Neoral) (mainly limited to management of membranous nephritis)

For vasculitis
- cyclophosphamide
- methotrexate
- azathioprine

GENERAL CONCEPTS OF DMARD USE

Treatment with conventional and biologic DMARDs is best done in partnership with a rheumatologist or other expert clinician.

- Ensure that the diagnosis is clear and indications are appropriate for the DMARD choice.

- Decide on the end points that will indicate treatment success or failure (clinical parameters, biomarkers, etc.).

- Review with the patient drug interactions and the side-effect profile of the chosen DMARD.

- Discuss pregnancy risks, contraception, and fertility with female patients and couples.

- Organize appropriate screening blood work and/or urinalysis and other necessary testing for baseline and regular monitoring for drug toxicity. Routinely remind patients about adherence to safety monitoring.

- Patients with rheumatic diseases are at increased risk for developing vaccine-preventable infections, which can lead to significant morbidity and mortality. If possible, appropriate vaccinations (hepatitis B, pneumococcal vaccine, influenza vaccine, varicella and herpes zoster vaccine in older adults) should be done before initiation of immunosuppressive therapy. In patients where this is not possible, up-to-date recommendations (from rheumatology and infectious disease societies) should be used to guide the vaccination schedule.

BIOLOGICS

- The introduction of biologic DMARDs has resulted in significantly improved outcomes in patients with rheumatoid arthritis (and an increasing list of other diseases).
- These drugs have created the capacity to achieve a state of true remission, or at least very low disease activity in many patients.
- The list of biologic response modifiers and their indications is rapidly evolving (see Table 12.3 for current information).
- These drugs are extremely expensive: patients usually require supplemental coverage (e.g., through insurance plans, or special government plans).

Indications

- The indication for therapy with biologic agents is generally failure of conventional DMARDs and immunosuppressive agents.
- An exception is management of inflammatory spondylitis. It is recommended that patients

Therapeutics

TABLE 12.3. Commonly used biologic agents: mechanism of action and side effects

Mode of action		Drug	Administration/ Frequency	Indications
TNFα inhibitor	Anti-TNFα: chimeric mAb	Infliximab	IV every 6–8 weeks after initial loading dose (0, 2, 6 weeks)	RA, PsA, AS
	Anti-TNFα: human mAb	Adalimumab	SC every 2 weeks	
	Anti-TNFα: human mAb	Golimumab	SC every 4 weeks	
	Soluble TNF receptor-Fc construct	Etanercept	SC weekly	RA, PsA, AS
	Humanized PEGylated Fab' fragment	Certolizumab	SC every 2 weeks or every 4 weeks after initial injections at 0, 2, and 4 weeks	
Costimulation inhibitor	Soluble CTLA-4-Ig (Fc) construct	Abatacept	IV once monthly or SC once weekly	RA (??SLE)
Interleukin-6 receptor inhibitor	Humanized mAb against IL6R	Tocilizumab	IV every 4 weeks or SC every 2 weeks	RA, Still disease, JIA
B-cell depletion	Chimeric mAb against CD20	Rituximab	Once weekly × 2 doses (RA), may be retreated at 6 months; different protocols for other diseases	RA, GPA, inflammatory myositis (?), others
Inhibition of B-cell survival	mAb against BLyS, a B-cell survival factor	Belimumab	IV every 4 weeks after loading dose	SLE (not renal or CNS disease)

Abbreviations: AS, ankylosing spondylitis; CTLA-4, cytotoxic T-lymphocyte-associated antigen 4; GPA, granulomatosis with polyangiitis; IL6R, interleukin 6 receptor; JIA, juvenile idiopathic arthritis; mAb, monoclonal antibody; PsA, psoriatic arthritis; RA, rheumatoid arthritis; SC, subcutaneously; SLE, systemic lupus erythematosus; TNFα, tumour necrosis factor alpha.

failing therapy with NSAIDs be offered therapy with an anti-TNF agent, as conventional DMARDs do not work for this clinical problem.

- Indications for introducing biologics, and the timing of their introduction, will continue to evolve.

Side effects

The side effects of most biologic agents are similar. They include:

Infection: This is the most common adverse reaction with all biologics studied.

- There is an increased risk for serious infections, including bacterial infections, tuberculosis (especially reactivation of latent tuberculosis), reactivation of hepatitis B, and opportunistic infections.
- With anti-B cell therapy (rituximab), there has been concern for reactivation of JC virus causing progressive multifocal leukoencephalopathy (PML).

Cytopenias: Infrequently, neutropenia and thrombocytopenia have been described (more frequent with anti-IL-6 therapy).

Hepatotoxicity: This is more frequent with anti-IL-6 therapy.

GI perforation: Concern for this complication is associated with anti-IL-6 therapy, especially in those with diverticular disease.

Malignancy: Long-term follow-up of TNF inhibitors to date has not demonstrated a higher rate of malignancies, except for nonmelanoma skin cancers. Ongoing surveillance will be required for all biologic agents.

Neurologic effects: Rare development or worsening of demyelination (anti-TNF therapy) can occur.

Cardiovascular effects: Congestive heart failure can occur with anti-TNF therapy. Increased cholesterol levels can occur with anti-IL-6 therapy.

Immunologic effects: Development of anticardiolipin, antinuclear, and anti-dsDNA antibodies can occur (though clinical drug-induced lupus is rare).

Therapeutics

Infusion reactions: Patients may have minor local reactions with subcutaneous injections, or more severe systemic reactions with IV agents. Some infusions call for GC premedication.

Patients should have screening for tuberculosis (skin test, chest X-ray) and hepatitis B (serology) before initiating biologic therapy (also see comments in "General Concepts of DMARD Use" regarding immunizations).

MONITORING

- Monitoring includes regular evaluation of liver enzymes, CBC, and lipid profile (for certain agents).

- Patients should discontinue their biologic agent if they develop an intercurrent infection, particularly if antibiotics are required.

- Temporary discontinuation before surgical procedures is generally recommended (agents should be discontinued at least 1 week before surgery, but longer intervals may be appropriate depending on the half-life of the biologic agent, the nature of the surgery, and the patient's condition).

- Biologics may be restarted postoperatively if there is no evidence of infection and if wound healing is progressing well.

Further Reading

Coursin DB, Wood KE. Corticosteroid supplementation for adrenal insufficiency. *JAMA.* 2002;287(2):236–40. http://dx.doi.org/10.1001/jama.287.2.236. Medline:11779267

Harirforoosh S, Asghar W, Jamali F. Adverse effects of nonsteroidal antiinflammatory drugs: an update of gastrointestinal, cardiovascular and renal complications. *J Pharm Pharm Sci.* 2013;16(5):821–47. Medline:24393558

Rhen T, Cidlowski JA. Antiinflammatory action of glucocorticoids—new mechanisms for old drugs. *N Engl J Med.* 2005;353(16):1711–23. http://dx.doi.org/10.1056/NEJMra050541. Medline:16236742

Timlin H, Bingham CO III. Efficacy and safety implications of molecular constructs of biological agents for rheumatoid arthritis. *Expert Opin Biol Ther.* 2014;14(7):893–904. http://dx.doi.org/10.1517/14712598.2014.900536. Medline:24720727

SECTION 4: SELECTED RHEUMATOLOGIC EMERGENCIES

13

Septic Arthritis, Osteomyelitis, Septic Bursitis, and Tenosynovitis

DR. REGINA M. TAYLOR-GJEVRE
UNIVERSITY OF SASKATCHEWAN

These clinical presentations are often seen in patients in the emergency department and in those admitted to general medical wards. It is therefore crucial to be able to recognize, evaluate, and treat these serious conditions. Septic arthritis is an **emergency** in rheumatology.

SEPTIC ARTHRITIS

KEY CONCEPTS: SEPTIC ARTHRITIS

1. Consider the possibility of infection in any inflamed joint.
2. Arthrocentesis and synovial fluid analysis are **essential** for diagnosis and should not be delayed when there is a strong clinical suspicion for septic arthritis.
3. Septic arthritis may be categorized as gonococcal and nongonococcal.
4. Septic arthritis requires urgent initiation of antibiotics, as well as drainage of the joint.
5. Failure to diagnose and treat may lead to irreversible joint destruction and death.
6. Orthopedic consultation should be considered early in the course, particularly in cases of suspected hip infection, prosthetic joint infection, or joints that are technically

difficult to drain. A collaborative multidisciplinary approach may also be desired in patients with complex presentations involving structurally abnormal or previously damaged joints, multiple comorbidities, and/or immunocompromised states.

History: Septic Arthritis

PATIENT DEMOGRAPHICS

Septic arthritis can occur at any age, but children and the elderly are more likely to present with it. Other predisposing risk factors include:

Comorbidities associated with impaired immune function:

- These include systemic diseases: diabetes mellitus, liver disease, alcoholism, malignancies, and chronic kidney disease, particularly hemodialysis-dependent patients.
- Intravenous drug use is also relevant.

Use of immunosuppressive medications:

- Consider disease-modifying antirheumatic drugs (DMARDs), glucocorticoids, and biologics in patients with preexisting rheumatic diseases.
- Transplant patients and others on chronic immunomodulatory therapy are also at risk.

Structural abnormalities in the joint that predispose to infection: These include prosthetic joints, Charcot joints, previous joint injury, or arthritic involvement such as in rheumatoid arthritis.

Opportunities for introduction of infection:

- These include recent joint surgery; intra-articular joint injection (estimated 1 to 4 cases per 10 000 injections); concurrent extra-articular infection with potential for local (e.g., cellulitis) or hematogenous spread (e.g., endocarditis or other causes of bacteremia) to joints.

- Exposure through sexual activity is also relevant: up to 3% of patients with untreated gonococcal mucosal infections develop disseminated gonococcal infection (DGI).

KEY QUESTIONS: SEPTIC ARTHRITIS

1. What is the nature of the joint involvement and distribution?

- The typical presentation of acute septic arthritis is a history of acute pain and swelling in a single joint. The knee and hip are the most common sites; however, any joint may be involved. The infection may be polyarticular in 15% of cases.

- In neonates and infants, septic arthritis may be deceptive. The classic signs of infection may be absent. A high index of suspicion and careful examination are particularly required in these age groups.

- An atypical presentation with a more insidious onset and subtler symptoms may occur in elderly and immunocompromised patients.

- Atypical locations for septic arthritis such as the SI or sternoclavicular joints are more commonly seen among IV drug users.

- People with chronic arthritis such as rheumatoid arthritis have a tenfold higher risk of septic arthritis. This may manifest as a single joint with disproportionate inflammation, or excess pain and swelling compared with other joints affected by the chronic arthritis. A high index of suspicion is required.

- In gonococcal arthritis, there are 2 clinical presentations: a "bacteremic" form that includes migratory polyarthralgia or polyarthritis, tenosynovitis, and dermatitis, and a "suppurative" form in which arthritis (usually a monoarthritis) is the main feature. Knees, wrists, ankles, and fingers are the most commonly affected joints.

2. Have there been any recent exposures or potential portals of entry?

Inquire about trauma, surgery, and recent or current infections (GU, pulmonary, skin).

3. What is the social history?

- Ask about sexual activity and risk of exposure, as well as symptoms of sexually transmitted disease.

  - In women, particularly, the initial mucosal infection may be relatively asymptomatic. DGI is 4 times more common in women than men and is more likely to develop during menstruation or pregnancy.

- Is there a history of IV drug use?

4. Are there other medical conditions?

- Inquire particularly about conditions that suppress immune function (diabetes mellitus; chronic liver disease or cirrhosis; chronic kidney disease; dialysis).

- Is there a preexisting arthritis? A history of joint damage or surgery? A prosthetic joint?

5. Are any medications being taken?

- Are there any immunosuppressive medications being used, especially glucocorticoids?

- Has there been any recent antibiotic use that might affect culture results?

Physical Examination: Septic Arthritis

Vital signs:

- Most patients have fever, although it may be low grade (less than 39°C).

- Elderly or immunocompromised hosts may be less able to mount a febrile response.

- Patients typically appear unwell.

General examination:

- There may be extra-articular sites of infection associated with septic arthritis.
- Examine the skin for evidence of pustules such as seen in DGI dermatitis.
- Look for signs of infection at a previous IV access site or a cellulitis.
- Examine the patient for evidence of concurrent endocarditis or pneumonia.
- Assess features of GU tract infections. Urethritis or cervicitis may be found in gonococcal disease.

Musculoskeletal examination:

- Note whether the involved joint is native or prosthetic. Is there evidence of underlying arthritis? Are other joints inflamed?
- Septic joints are effused and usually warm to the touch. The joint may be erythematous. A septic joint will be very painful and accordingly will have a restricted range of motion.

Key Laboratory Investigations: Septic Arthritis

CBC: This may show an increased WBC count with left shift.

Acute phase reactants: These will be elevated, including ESR and CRP.

Creatinine, liver enzymes: These provide a useful baseline; changes may reflect more severe infection.

Blood cultures:

- Obtain blood before starting antibiotic therapy to optimize the opportunity to identify the pathologic organism.

- Results are positive in 50% of nongonococcal arthritis; this percentage is likely lower in DGI cases.

Synovial fluid:

- Use an 18-gauge needle to aspirate septic joints, as pus may be thick!

- If you cannot aspirate the joint, consult rheumatology or orthopedics urgently.

- Deep joints such as the hip or SI joint should be aspirated by radiology under fluoroscopic guidance.

- **WBC in synovial fluid:** This is often greater than $50\,000 \times 10^6$/L, with less than 75% neutrophils (typically less than 90%).

- **Synovial fluid Gram stain and culture:** Definitive diagnosis of septic arthritis requires identification of bacteria in the synovial fluid or on subsequent culture. **Cultures must be obtained without delay.** With increased concerns around microbial resistance, collection of culture materials before antibiotic initiation allows the best chance to provide targeted therapy based on the antimicrobial susceptibilities of the specific organism.

- Gram stain is positive in 50% of nongonococcal cases, and cultures are positive in 67% of cases. There may be greater yield on culture with inoculation of joint fluid into blood culture bottles.

  - With gonococcal arthritis, approximately 50% of synovial fluid cultures are positive. Less than half of the culture-positive gonococcal specimens have positive direct Gram stains.

- In suspected gonococcal arthritis, collect urethral cultures (positive in 90% of infected men), cultures from the uterine endocervix (positive in 50% to 70% of infected women), or urine samples for nucleic acid testing. Rectal and pharyngeal cultures have lower positivity rates.

- Polymerase chain reaction techniques may detect *Neisseria gonorrhoeae* DNA even when cultures are negative.

CAUTIONS ON LABORATORY INVESTIGATIONS IN SEPTIC ARTHRITIS

- Ten percent of cases are never confirmed with blood or synovial fluid cultures.

- In patients with underlying crystalline arthritis (gout or calcium pyrophosphate dihydrate crystal deposition), crystals may be present in the synovial fluid concurrently with an infection. The presence of crystals on microscopic examination does **not** rule out septic arthritis.

- Mycobacterial and fungal arthritis are much less common than bacterial arthritis, but can be seen in the setting of immunosuppression. An indolent monoarthritis is often the only symptom, and synovial membrane histopathological analysis and culture are frequently required to establish the diagnosis.

Imaging: Septic Arthritis

Plain radiographs: This should be the first imaging technique used and will provide a baseline. Most often, radiographs appear normal in the initial stages. Subsequently, osteopenia may be evident. In later stages, diffuse joint-space narrowing may evolve.

Ultrasound: This may be helpful in detecting joint effusions and permit performance of guided diagnostic arthrocentesis.

CT imaging: This is a superior technique for visualization of bone edema, erosions, osteitic foci, and sclerosis. It may also help to confirm the presence of effusion in difficult-to-examine joints such as hip or SI joints.

MRI: This is the preferred imaging technique for differentiating bone and soft-tissue involvement.

Radionuclide scans: These may be used to localize areas of inflammation.

Differential Diagnosis: Septic Arthritis

See chapter 1.

Initial Approach to Treatment: Septic Arthritis

- Treatment involves early initiation of antibiotics (immediately after cultures are sent) and prompt debridement for removal of purulent infected material.

- Needle aspiration may be used as an initial method of joint drainage and may be required 1 time to several times daily. If needle aspiration is technically difficult, proving inadequate, or the effusion continues to reaccumulate for more than 7 days, arthroscopy and open drainage may be required. Orthopedic consultation early in the course of septic arthritis is often advisable.

- Early antibiotic treatment should be based on the clinical presentation, the most likely organism to be involved (see Table 13.1), and direct Gram stain results. Start antibiotics immediately following collection of culture materials (see Table 13.2). Antibiotic choices may then be adjusted once culture and susceptibility results are available.

TABLE 13.1. Organisms associated with septic arthritis

Organism	Clinical clues	Risk group
Staphylococcus aureus This is the most common organism	This is the most common organism	MRSA is often more virulent than MSSA infections
	It may be associated with cellulitis, endocarditis, abscesses, IV drug abuse	
	MRSA is increasing in IV drug use, elderly patients, and orthopedic-associated infection, including prosthetic joints	
Coagulase-negative staphylococci	This is the most common contaminant in synovial fluid cultures	Patients with prosthetic joints are at risk
Streptococci		
ß-hemolytic groups A, B, C, G; *Streptococcus pneumoniae*	Look for recent streptococcal infection such as pneumonia	Patients are often immunocompromised
Gram-negative organisms	These occur in 5%–20% of cases	This is primarily seen in children, immunosuppressed patients, IV drug users
	They may be associated with concurrent UTIs	Salmonella may be seen in patients receiving anti-TNF therapies and in patients with sickle cell disease
Neisseria gonorrhoeae	Look for arthralgias or arthritis; tenosynovitis; dermatitis	Patients are sexually active, often young healthy adults
Pasteurella multocida	Look for cat bite	This is often associated with osteomyelitis
TB, fungal	Look for chronic monoarthritis	Risk group includes HIV population, individuals from endemic areas, immunosuppressed individuals

Abbreviations: MRSA, methicillin-resistant *Staphylococcus aureus*; MSSA, methicillin-sensitive *Staphylococcus aureus*; TB, tuberculosis; TNF, tumour necrosis factor; UTIs, urinary tract infections.

TABLE 13.2. Initial empiric antibiotic choices for septic arthritis

Clinical scenario	Antibiotic choice	Comments
Young sexually active person in whom gonococcal infection is suspected	Ceftriaxone 1 g IV q24 hours Doxycycline 100 mg po bid × 7 days or single-dose azithromycin 1 g to cover possible concurrent chlamydia infection	Duration of therapy should be 7–14 days of ceftriaxone Partner(s) should be treated concurrently
Any age, gonococcal infection not suspected	Cloxacillin 2 g IV q4–6h or cefazolin 1–2 g IV q8h	If MRSA is a possibility, consider use of vancomycin
Gram-positive organism on direct stain	Cefazolin 1–2 g IV q8h	If MRSA is a possibility, consider use of vancomycin
Gram-negative organism on direct stain	Antipseudomonal cephalosporin (e.g., cefepime 2 g IV q12h or ceftazidime 1–2 g IV q8h) or an anti-pseudomonal carbapenem	4 weeks of parenteral therapy is recommended for gram-negative septic arthritis

Abbreviations: bid, twice a day; MRSA, methicillin-resistant *Staphylococcus aureus*; po, orally; q, every.

- Repeated synovial fluid analysis should demonstrate decreasing cell counts and negative culture results if the antibiotic choice is appropriate.
- Duration of therapy for nongonococcal septic arthritis is 2 to 4 weeks of parenteral therapy with a subsequent course of oral therapy. Recommendations on duration of IV versus oral therapy vary, depending on the organism. The course of therapy may need to be prolonged to optimally manage infection with particular pathogens, and in patients with implants or infections involving other sites (e.g., infective endocarditis).
- Early consultation of allied health professionals, physical therapists, and occupational therapists

for both splinting and preservation of range of motion is advisable.

- When possible, discontinue any immunosuppressive medications the patient may be taking. **Caution**: This does not apply to patients taking glucocorticoids on a longer-term basis, as they may have adrenal suppression. These patients will not be able to discontinue this medication safely and may in some cases require stress dosing.

OSTEOMYELITIS

KEY CONCEPTS: OSTEOMYELITIS

1. Osteomyelitis is an inflammation of the bone and bone marrow usually caused by bacteria. Infection is caused by bacteria that gain access to bone, either hematogenously via direct spread from a contiguous focus of infection or from a local injury site.
2. Osteomyelitis may be categorized as acute (before development of necrotic bone) or chronic (with development of necrotic bone, termed *sequestrum*).
3. Diagnosis may be challenging. Consider the possibility in any patient with fever and bony discomfort.
4. Definitive diagnosis is based on bone biopsy and culture.
5. An orthopedic and infectious disease consultation as part of a multidisciplinary approach is often optimal.

History: Osteomyelitis

- Predisposing factors include open fractures, malnutrition, malignancy, chronic alcoholism, smoking, diabetes mellitus, IV drug use, hemodialysis, and immunosuppression (e.g., chronic glucocorticoid use).
- Hematogenous spread affects the spine (lumbar more than thoracic more than cervical), pelvis,

and small bones preferentially. Long bone involvement in adults is generally associated with open fractures.

- Symptoms of acute osteomyelitis include acute febrile illness with localized discomfort and tenderness. Typically, swelling and erythema are present over the affected region. **Caution:** Patients with neuropathies (e.g., diabetics) may report little pain.

- A history of a recent infection may identify the focus source for the osteomyelitis. A thorough review of systems to search for infections will be required. **Caution:** A spinal epidural abscess may complicate vertebral osteomyelitis, presenting as progressive spinal pain.

- Chronic osteomyelitis may present with nonspecific symptoms, which may be intermittent and recurring. Weight loss and malaise may be reported.

Physical Examination: Osteomyelitis

- There may be little to find on examination. The area affected may exhibit adjacent swelling or erythema. There may be tenderness to palpation around the site of osteomyelitis.

- A careful complete physical examination is necessary to evaluate potential portals of entry for infection, including areas of trauma, skin infection, or breakdown such as decubitus ulcers.

- Diabetic or rheumatoid foot ulcers extending to bone should be considered to have associated osteomyelitis.

Key Laboratory Investigations: Osteomyelitis

Acute osteomyelitis: There is an acute phase response with increased ESR and CRP. There is usually a mild increase in WBC count.

Chronic osteomyelitis: Sixty-five percent of patients have elevated ESR and/or CRP; however, the WBC count is often normal.

Blood cultures: Results may be positive in acute osteomyelitis.

- **Microbiology:** See Table 13.3.

TABLE 13.3. Microbiology in osteomyelitis

Mechanism	Organisms	Notes	Population	Empiric antibiotics
Hematogenous	*Staphylococcus aureus*, ß-hemolytic streptococci, enteric gram-negative rods	Infection generally involves a single organism It often occurs in axial sites in adults, and long bones in children	Children and people over age 50	MRSA coverage: use vancomycin MSSA coverage: use cefazolin or cloxacillin Additional coverage for gram-negative rods may be required
Contiguous focus	*S. aureus*, *Streptococcus pyogenes*, *Enterococcus* spp., gram-negative rods, anaerobes	Polymicrobial		See notes for hematogenous infection, above A choice for coverage of gram-negative rods and anaerobes may be piperacillin-tazobactam
Vascular insufficiency related	*S. aureus*, *Streptococcus* sp., enteric gram-negative bacilli, *Pseudomonas aeruginosa*, anaerobes	Polymicrobial		Piperacillin-tazobactam

Abbreviations: MRSA, methicillin-resistant *Staphylococcus aureus*; MSSA, methicillin-sensitive *Staphylococcus aureus*.

Imaging: Osteomyelitis

A definitive diagnosis requires a bone biopsy. No noninvasive test can definitely establish a diagnosis of osteomyelitis. However, imaging consistent with osteomyelitis in the setting of a positive blood culture is highly suggestive and is considered by many clinicians to be sufficient for the diagnosis.

Plain films: These should be taken as a first step. They may suggest the correct diagnosis, exclude other pathological conditions, and serve as a baseline. Bone destruction and periosteal reaction will be present only after 1 to 2 weeks. In chronic osteomyelitis, bone sclerosis, periosteal new bone formation, and sequestra are seen.

Three-phase bone scan: This is a useful screening test. It includes an initial flow phase, blood pool phase (10 minutes), and delayed static imaging (3 hours). In cellulitis, the first 2 phases show increased uptake. By contrast, osteomyelitis reveals intense uptake in all 3 phases. This scan is useful for detecting multifocal involvement.

Gallium scan: This is more specific, but less sensitive, than a bone scan. The combination of a bone and gallium scan in some centres may be helpful. It is always best to speak to your local nuclear medicine physicians if in doubt.

WBC scan: This may be better at determining whether inflammation is within the bone, but it is not always available.

CT scan: This can be used to evaluate focal findings, but is less sensitive than bone scan and MRI.

MRI:

- This is the test of choice, if available. It is extremely sensitive in the early detection of osteomyelitis. It is also excellent for visualizing soft tissues, which may contain an abscess.

- MRI of the spine is essential for evaluation of vertebral osteomyelitis and to assess for a spinal epidural abscess. This clinical presentation requires urgent assessment and intervention.

Open bone biopsy: This is the gold standard. It can begin with needle biopsy and, if required, progress to an open biopsy.

Treatment: Osteomyelitis

- If acute osteomyelitis is not treated adequately, chronic osteomyelitis may result, which is more challenging to treat.
- Antibiotics should be started **only after** appropriate cultures have been sent (as long as the patient is stable). A specific microbiological diagnosis is essential.
- Organisms isolated from sinus tract drainage may not accurately reflect organisms present in the bone. If blood cultures are negative, do a bone biopsy before empiric antibiotics. If the patient appears toxic, you may need to treat before bone biopsy, but in more indolent presentations, it is better to establish a definitive microbiological diagnosis.
- The final choice of antibiotics will be adjusted on the basis of culture results. Table 13.3 lists empiric choices.
- Usually 6 or more weeks of IV antibiotic treatment is required. Some centres will complete therapy with oral antibiotics in selected patients.
- Surgical consultation should be considered, especially for patients who are not responding to antibiotics after 48 hours, or who have a soft tissue abscess (including epidural abscess), a concomitant joint infection, or instability of the spine.
- Consider infectious disease consultation.

SEPTIC BURSITIS

KEY CONCEPTS: SEPTIC BURSITIS

1. Superficial bursae most frequently become infected by direct percutaneous traumatic inoculation of pathogens or by contiguous spread from an adjacent infection such as a cellulitis. The most common sites of involvement are the olecranon and the prepatellar bursae.

2. By contrast, infection of deep bursae, such as the subacromial bursa, is often related to either hematogenous spread or complications from a local injection.

3. Clinical features include erythema, swelling, and tenderness.

4. *Staphylococcus aureus* is the most common isolate in more than 80% of cases, followed in frequency by group B hemolytic streptococci and then enterococci, gram-negative rods, and coagulase-negative *Staphylococcus* spp.

5. In chronic bursitis, atypical organisms such as mycobacteria, *Brucella*, or fungi may need to be considered.

6. The differential diagnosis includes gouty and traumatic bursitis.

7. Bursal fluid aspiration and/or drainage and examination for crystals, Gram stain, and culture are essential.

8. Empiric antibiotics should be initiated early, targeting staphylococci and streptococci, and then adjusted as culture results become available.

9. If a patient does not respond to therapy, surgical consultation may be advisable.

SEPTIC TENOSYNOVITIS

KEY CONCEPTS: SEPTIC TENOSYNOVITIS

1. The flexor tendons and digital tendon sheaths of the hands are the most common sites for septic tenosynovitis.

2. Local sequelae include necrosis and tendon rupture.

3. The 4 cardinal signs of septic flexor hand tenosynovitis are:

- uniform symmetric finger swelling
- digit held in partial flexion at rest
- tenderness to palpation along length of tendon sheath
- pain along the tendon sheath with passive digit extension

4. It most commonly follows local trauma; less frequently, it may be attributable to hematogenous spread.

5. The most common causative organisms include *S. aureus*, *S. epidermidis*, streptococci, enterococci, and gram-negative rods. Bite wounds are often polymicrobial. In cases of *N. gonorrhea* infection, tenosynovitis is common.

6. The gold standard for diagnosis is culture of synovial sheath fluid.

7. Timely empiric antibiotics should be initiated, based on the nature of injury and history, and then adjusted accordingly when culture results become available.

8. Early surgical consultation regarding the need for operative intervention should be considered.

9. Mycobacterial or fungal infections need to be considered in cases of chronic tenosynovitis.

Acknowledgement

Thanks to Dr. Susan Humphrey-Murto, University of Ottawa, who developed this chapter for the first edition of the *Canadian Residents' Rheumatology Handbook*, 2005.

Further Reading

García-Arias M, Balsa A, Mola EM. Septic arthritis. *Best Pract Res Clin Rheumatol*. 2011;25(3):407–21. http://dx.doi.org/10.1016/j.berh.2011.02.001. Medline:22100289

Mouzopoulos G, Kanakaris NK, Kontakis G, et al. Management of bone infections in adults: the surgeon's and microbiologist's perspectives. *Injury*. 2011;42(Suppl 5):S18–23. http://dx.doi.org/10.1016/S0020-1383(11)70128-0. Medline:22196905

Santiago Restrepo C, Giménez CR, McCarthy K. Imaging of osteomyelitis and musculoskeletal soft tissue infections: current concepts. *Rheum Dis Clin North Am*. 2003;29(1):89–109. http://dx.doi.org/10.1016/S0889-857X(02)00078-9. Medline:12635502

Sharff KA, Richards EP, Townes JM. Clinical management of septic arthritis. *Curr Rheumatol Rep*. 2013;15(6):332. http://dx.doi.org/10.1007/s11926-013-0332-4. Medline:23591823

Torralba KD, Quismorio FP Jr. Soft tissue infections. *Rheum Dis Clin North Am*. 2009;35(1):45–62. http://dx.doi.org/10.1016/j.rdc.2009.03.002. Medline:19480996

14

Giant Cell Arteritis

DR. DAVID B. ROBINSON
UNIVERSITY OF MANITOBA

KEY CONCEPTS

1. Giant cell arteritis (GCA) is the most common systemic vasculitis in North America.
2. An idiopathic large vessel vasculitis, it affects the second to fifth branches of the aorta.
3. Individuals 50 years of age and over are affected, with increased incidence after age 70.
4. There is a high overlap with polymyalgia rheumatica (PMR).
5. Clinical manifestations arise from ischemia in the affected tissues in combination with constitutional symptoms arising from circulating cytokines.
6. There are several distinct clinical patterns with which patients can present.
7. Urgent diagnosis and treatment is required to prevent abrupt onset of irreversible blindness in a small number of cases.

History

PATIENT DEMOGRAPHICS

- GCA occurs almost exclusively in individuals older than 50 years, but more commonly in 70- to 80-year-olds.

- Prevalence is highest in those of northern European descent.

KEY QUESTIONS

Giant cell arteritis can present with several distinct clinical patterns. There are 4 major patterns, but combinations of findings can occur. It is most useful to organize questions to identify 1 of the patterns. Diagnosis often requires a careful history and physical examination, and it is often difficult.

1. Are there cranial artery symptoms?

- **Headache:** New-onset headache or new pattern of headache in elderly patients should prompt consideration of GCA. Patients may have scalp tenderness or discomfort noted when combing their hair, wearing hats, or lying down with pressure on their scalp.

- **Jaw claudication:** Patients may have discomfort in their temporalis or masseter muscles, or tongue discomfort while talking or chewing. This is usually relieved with rest, similar to claudication in the legs in peripheral vascular disease.

- **Visual changes:** Abrupt visual loss may occur because of involvement of the posterior ciliary or ophthalmic arteries supplying the optic nerve. The visual loss is often irreversible. Visual loss in 1 eye raises the risk of loss in the other. This can usually be prevented by prompt and adequate therapy.

- **Stroke:** Intracranial vessels are usually spared because of lack of an internal elastic lamina. Case reports of stroke due to occlusion of carotid arteries do exist. The exact incidence of stroke in GCA is impossible to determine because of lack of tissue for pathological analysis and a high incidence of atheroembolic strokes in this age group.

2. Is there involvement of the aorta or primary branches?

- Severe stenosis in the subclavian, carotid, and axillary arteries occurs in 10% to 15% of patients with GCA.

- Symptoms at presentation include limb claudication, paresthesias, ischemic changes, and new-onset Raynaud phenomenon. Cranial symptoms are frequently absent. The results of temporal artery biopsies are usually negative in the absence of cranial symptoms. Constitutional symptoms may be absent.

3. Are there symptoms of polymyalgia rheumatica (PMR)?

- PMR is extremely common in individuals over 50 years of age and is considered by many to be part of a spectrum of disease with GCA.

- It follows or precedes GCA in 40% to 60% of cases, and all patients with PMR should be watched for development of GCA.

- Clinically, patients present with aching and pain in the neck, pectoral, and pelvic girdles.

- Symptoms are often worse at night and patients describe difficulty turning over in bed with prolonged morning stiffness. Constitutional symptoms of fatigue and malaise are often present.

- There is no specific diagnostic test. Acute phase reactants are usually elevated.

- Near complete relief with glucocorticoids (prednisone 15–20 mg) occurs within hours and helps confirm diagnosis.

4. Is this a fever of unknown origin?

- GCA may account for a significant proportion of fever of unknown origin in patients over 65 years of age.

- In these cases, arteritis occurs without vessel lumen narrowing and tissue ischemia.
- Fever, malaise, weight loss, and night sweats can occur in isolation or in conjunction with 1 of the presentations described above.

Physical Examination

Each of the clinical presentations above has different physical manifestations that should be sought on examination.

Cranial arteries:
- Check for scalp tenderness; masseter and temporalis tenderness; temporal artery thickening, tenderness, or pulselessness.
- Funduscopy may be normal or may show pallor or edema of the optic disc, "cotton wool" patches, or small hemorrhages.

Large vessels:
- Check BP in both arms and pulses in all limbs.
- Look for peripheral signs of tissue ischemia.
- Listen for bruits over large vessels and palpate for an aortic aneurysm.

Joints: The source of myalgias in PMR may be related to bursitis in the pectoral and pelvic girdle, giving severe discomfort on palpation and range of motion.

Other:
- Always try to elicit alternative causes for the patient's symptoms during the physical examination (and history).
- In this age group, malignancy and indolent infections can present with chronic constitutional symptoms.
- Atherosclerosis may cause ischemic symptoms without elevations in inflammatory markers.

Key Laboratory Investigations

ESR and CRP:

- Highly elevated ESRs are usually found in GCA. CRP is also elevated and is more specific for the acute phase response than ESR.
- Anemia of chronic disease and thrombocytosis are also common.
- GCA can occur infrequently with normal acute phase reactants.

Temporal artery biopsy:

- A definite diagnosis of GCA requires pathological examination of arterial tissue.
- Temporal artery biopsy is a minimally invasive procedure with few adverse effects.
- The presence of jaw claudication, diplopia, and an enlarged temporal artery are predictive of a positive biopsy result. Conversely, patients with aortitis and no cranial symptoms are unlikely to have a positive biopsy result.
- Because of the presence of skip lesions, a 2- to 3-cm specimen of temporal artery should be obtained. A bilateral temporal artery biopsy is rarely helpful and not recommended.
- Biopsy results may be positive after several weeks of steroid therapy but the yield declines with time.
  - Biopsies should be obtained as early as possible while not delaying steroid treatment.
  - While it is tempting in certain cases to forgo biopsy, it can be invaluable further on in treatment if the patient develops atypical symptoms or has a poor response to treatment.
  - A biopsy should be performed whenever possible.

- **Pathology on biopsy:** Biopsy may show panarteritis with giant cell granuloma formation. Also look for disruption of internal elastic lamina and intimal thickening. Involvement may be patchy and skip lesions are seen.

Imaging

CRANIAL VESSELS

- For evaluation of cranial vessels, there is no modality sufficiently robust to replace temporal artery biopsy and none are in widespread use.
- **Ultrasonography** of the temporal arteries may yield a typical "halo" sign, which has fair specificity for GCA, but is operator dependent.

GCA WITH LARGE VESSEL INVOLVEMENT

Imaging has far more value in patients with large vessel involvement.

- **Conventional X-ray angiography** may show typical stenotic lesions of the subclavian, axillary, proximal brachial, or carotid arteries.
- Aortitis leads to dilatation and aneurysm formation. **Computed tomography angiography (CTA)** may be helpful by demonstrating vessel wall thickening. **MRI** or **magnetic resonance angiography (MRA)** may also show vessel wall edema suggestive of inflammation. There is some concern that MRI and MRA may over diagnose inflammation in some cases.
- **^{18}F-fluorodeoxyglucose (FDG) positron emission tomography** can demonstrate increased metabolic activity associated with large vessel inflammation. It may not be helpful in following disease once treatment has started, as neovascularization may cause positive findings.

Initial Therapy

GLUCOCORTICOIDS

Glucocorticoids are the mainstay of therapy and should be instituted promptly to avoid vision loss.

- Usual therapy is with prednisone at 1 mg/kg of body weight until symptoms improve (usually 2 to 4 weeks) and then tapered by 10 mg per 1 to 2 weeks.
  - Once at 20 mg, tapering should be slower (2.5 mg per week), and slower still once 10 mg is reached (1 mg every 2 to 4 weeks).
  - Tapering regimens vary considerably.
  - Return of symptoms or elevation of acute phase reactants should prompt return to previous dose of steroid that controlled symptoms.
  - Elevation of acute phase reactants alone may not necessarily indicate need for increased steroid if the patient is clinically well. Avoid the knee-jerk reaction of increasing steroids on the basis of laboratory tests alone.
- Treatment may be prolonged and last several years in some patients.

STEROID-SPARING AGENTS

- Conflicting results have been obtained in trials using methotrexate as a steroid-sparing agent in GCA.
- Inconsistent results have also been found with several other immunosuppressives.
- Most clinicians use steroid-sparing agents in patients requiring unacceptably high steroid doses for symptom control.
- For methotrexate, it appears a minimum of 15 mg/wk is required for effect.
- Tocilizumab, a monoclonal antibody directed against the interleukin-6 receptor, may have a role in therapy of resistant disease.

PREVENTION OF COMPLICATIONS

- Patients should receive prophylaxis for osteoporosis in the form of calcium, vitamin D, and antiresorptive agents. Monitor for cognitive effects of steroids, hypertension, and diabetes mellitus.

- There appears to be an increased risk of thoracic aortic aneurysm as a late complication (up to 30%):
  - Given the advanced age and competing morbidities of this patient group, the most cost-effective screening protocol is not clear.
  - Annual chest radiography has been proposed by some authors.

Pitfalls in GCA Treatment

Problems often arise after patients have started therapy and either fail to respond or flare on fairly large doses of steroid. **Most of these questions arise in cases where a positive temporal artery biopsy result was not obtained.**

IS IT ALL ATHEROSCLEROSIS?
Ubiquitous in this age group, atherosclerotic lesions can mimic many of the symptoms of GCA. ESR may be falsely elevated or increased for other reasons.

IS THE ESR RELIABLE?
ESR may not reflect the acute phase response for several reasons. Normal ranges on laboratory sheets may not reflect the age-specific upper limit of normal (roughly half the patient's age). CRP may be more specific for inflammation than ESR.

WAS THE HEADACHE VASCULITIC?
Unfortunately, headaches stemming from several noninflammatory causes (e.g., migraine) may improve with glucocorticoids and a prompt response to prednisone is not always diagnostic.

Further Reading

García-Martínez A, Arguis P, Prieto-González S, et al. Prospective long term follow-up of a cohort of patients with giant cell arteritis screened for aortic structural damage (aneurysm or dilatation). *Ann Rheum Dis*. 2014;73(10):1826–32. http://dx.doi.org/10.1136/annrheumdis-2013-203322. Medline:23873881

Salvarani C, Pipitone N, Versari A, et al. Clinical features of polymyalgia rheumatica and giant cell arteritis. *Nat Rev Rheumatol*. 2012;8(9):509–21. http://dx.doi.org/10.1038/nrrheum.2012.97. Medline:22825731

Weyand CM, Goronzy JJ. Giant-cell arteritis and polymyalgia rheumatica. *Ann Intern Med*. 2003;139(6):505–15. http://dx.doi.org/10.7326/0003-4819-139-6-200309160-00015. Medline:13679329

Weyand CM, Goronzy JJ. Medium- and large-vessel vasculitis. *N Engl J Med*. 2003;349(2):160–9. http://dx.doi.org/10.1056/NEJMra022694. Medline:12853590

15

Pulmonary-Renal Syndromes

DR. ÉRIC RICH
UNIVERSITÉ DE MONTRÉAL

KEY CONCEPTS

1. Rapidly progressing glomerulonephritis and pulmonary infiltrates and/or hemorrhage define the pulmonary-renal syndromes that are often the manifestation of small vessel vasculitis.

2. The principal causative diseases are:

   - antineutrophil cytoplasmic antibody–associated vasculitis (ANCA-associated vasculitis): granulomatosis with polyangiitis (GPA), microscopic polyangiitis (MPA)
   - Goodpasture syndrome
   - connective tissue diseases such as systemic lupus erythematosus (SLE)

3. These patients need to be quickly recognized, thoroughly investigated, and aggressively treated as they may rapidly become critically ill.

4. Core diagnostic tests include CBC, creatinine, urinalysis, ANCA, antibodies to the glomerular basement membrane (anti-GBM), bronchoscopy, and organ biopsy (often kidney).

5. Intravenous methylprednisolone and cyclophosphamide, with or without plasmapheresis, should not be delayed: they should often be administered before confirmatory test results are available.

6. It is particularly important to establish efficient communication between the many specialties involved in the care of these patients (nephrologists, respirologists, rheumatologists, ICU physicians, radiologists).

History

- The combination of acute renal insufficiency and pulmonary infiltrates and/or hemorrhage can be seen in more common conditions such as: acute tubular necrosis accompanying severe pneumonia or acute respiratory distress syndrome; heart failure with prerenal impairment; any severe glomerular disease with marked fluid overload and pulmonary edema.

- If the clinical picture cannot be attributed to any of these more frequent causes, the possibility of small vessel vasculitis or connective tissue disease should be entertained.

- Lung capillaritis can lead to alveolar hemorrhage manifested by cough, severe dyspnea, and hemoptysis.

> *Pearl:* One-third of patients with diffuse alveolar hemorrhage will not have hemoptysis. In this case, dyspnea, diffuse pulmonary infiltrates, and decreasing hemoglobin levels will be your clues.

- Rapidly progressive glomerulonephritis may manifest with symptoms of uremia.

Pulmonary-renal syndrome can develop as a flare of an established disease or, more often, as the presenting feature of ANCA-associated vasculitis, Goodpasture syndrome, or connective tissue disease.

ANCA-ASSOCIATED VASCULITIS
- Intense arthralgias, fatigue, and low-grade fever are common to GPA and MPA.

- Unusually persistent sinusitis with nasal discharge, recurrent otitis, and red eyes are suggestive of GPA. Watch for stridor due to subglottic inflammation, because it can contribute to dyspnea and complicate ventilatory support in critically ill patients.
- Peripheral nerve involvement is seen in up to 50% of ANCA-associated vasculitis.
- Check for potential drug-induced vasculitis from treatment with propylthiouracil, minocycline, hydralazine, or allopurinol.

GOODPASTURE SYNDROME

Goodpasture syndrome is less frequent than ANCA-associated vasculitis.

> *Pearl:* Pulmonary hemorrhage occurs more frequently in current smokers. Goodpasture syndrome is usually associated with few preceding systemic symptoms.

CONNECTIVE TISSUE DISEASES

Look for SLE features (polyarthralgias, photosensitive rashes, serositis, etc.) and scleroderma (see chapter 5b).

OTHER RARE CAUSES

Other rare causes are other vasculitides (cryoglobulinemia, Henoch-Schönlein purpura), bacterial endocarditis, catastrophic antiphospholipid syndrome, thrombotic thrombocytopenic purpura, and hemolytic uremic syndrome.

Physical Examination

Vital signs:

- Fever should be a concern, because sepsis is a frequent mimicker or a superimposed complication.

Pul/renal syndrome

- Monitor oxygen saturation: patients can deteriorate rapidly and may require urgent transfer to ICU for ventilatory monitoring and support.

Eyes: Conjunctivitis, episcleritis, and scleritis are seen in ANCA-associated vasculitis and SLE.

Skin and mucous membranes:

- Subungual splinter hemorrhages and digital tip ischemic lesions are seen in ANCA-associated vasculitis, SLE, and infective endocarditis.
- Malar rash and shallow erythematous ulcers are seen on the hard palate in SLE.

Musculoskeletal exam: Some patients with ANCA-associated vasculitis and those with SLE may have inflammatory arthritis as part of their initial presentation.

Cardiorespiratory exam: Listen for stridor (GPA with upper airway involvement) and diffuse crackles. Usually there are no signs of pleural effusion.

Neurologic exam: Drop foot or wrist (due to mononeuritis multiplex) can be seen in ANCA-associated vasculitis.

Key Laboratory Investigations

INITIAL INVESTIGATIONS

CBC: Low and falling hemoglobin that is unexplained may indicate lung hemorrhage.

Creatinine: This is elevated in pulmonary-renal syndrome, or starting to trend upwards. Follow very carefully, even every 12 hours initially, because these patients can progress rapidly.

Urinalysis: This is essential and too often forgotten! Check daily for RBCs, RBC casts, and protein.

PTT/INR: Look for coagulation perturbation that may aggravate the condition.

Liver enzymes and alkaline phosphatase: These may be elevated.

Cultures of blood, urine, and/or sputum: Infection is a frequent comorbidity in these patients (and can also mimic pulmonary-renal syndrome).

ANCA:

- Confirm immunofluorescence results by enzyme-linked immunosorbent assay (this is essential); 90% of GPA patients are ANCA positive; cytoplasmic ANCA (cANCA)/anti-proteinase 3 (anti-PR3) are found in 85% of patients; and perinuclear ANCA (pANCA)/antimyeloperoxidase (anti-MPO) are found in the rest (see chapter 10).

- Seventy-five percent of patients with MPA are ANCA positive, almost exclusively pANCA/anti-MPO.

- Initially, ANCA can be negative in GPA limited to sinuses, but becomes positive when renal and/or lung involvement appears (up to 10% may remain ANCA negative).

Anti-GBM antibodies:

- In Goodpasture syndrome, 50% of patients have only kidney involvement and the other 50% both lung and renal disease.

- In 20% to 40% of anti-GBM-positive patients, ANCA will also be identified, more often pANCA/anti-MPO; disease in these "double positive" patients evolves more like ANCA-associated vasculitis.

Antinuclear antibodies (ANAs):

- Virtually all SLE patients are ANA positive; however, many unrelated conditions can have positive ANA (see chapter 10).

- Low serum complement levels (C3, C4) and elevated double-stranded DNA antibodies (anti-dsDNA) may help to support a diagnosis of SLE.

IMAGING AND OTHER PROCEDURES

Chest X-ray: Look for patchy or diffuse alveolar opacities.

Chest CT scan: Assess for alveolar ground-glass appearance (often central).

Pulmonary function tests: In pulmonary-renal syndromes, these show classically elevated diffusing capacity (DLCO) due to hemoglobin in the alveolar compartment. Patients are often too sick to do pulmonary function tests.

Bronchoscopy:

- Bronchoscopy is necessary to exclude infection in most cases.
- Bloody secretions are often seen in many lobes.
- Sequential bronchoalveolar lavage aspirates will show a progressive hemorrhagic return, suggestive of alveolar hemorrhage.
- Hemosiderin-laden macrophages will be identified when bleeding has been more chronic, and is helpful when overt hemorrhage is not seen despite alveolar infiltrates on X-rays.

BIOPSY

The high morbidity of the disease, the toxicity of therapies, and the need for long-term treatment make a firm diagnosis essential in pulmonary-renal syndromes. The gold standard is tissue biopsy of an affected organ. In severely ill patients, therapy may have to be initiated before a pathological diagnosis is available.

- Most often, the kidney is the preferred site to biopsy, as it is less risky than a lung biopsy in patients with limited respiratory reserve and is feasible even in patients on mechanical ventilation; specimens from a transbronchial lung biopsy are usually unsatisfactory and inconclusive.

- In GPA, a sinus biopsy is easily accessible, but diagnostic in only 25% of patients. A skin biopsy of "fresh" purpuric lesions will often show leukocytoclastic vasculitis, but will not permit differentiation among forms of vasculitis.

- A kidney biopsy of ANCA-associated vasculitis will show a characteristic pauci-immune necrotizing glomerulonephritis (i.e., scant or no immunoglobulins and/or complement on tissue immunofluorescence):

  - In Goodpasture syndrome, linear deposition of immunoglobulins along the basement membrane with crescentic glomerulonephritis is the standard finding.
  - In SLE, several patterns of immunoglobulin and/or complement deposition can be seen, with variable involvement of mesangium, glomerular capillaries, and crescent formation.

Initial Therapy

- Immunosuppression with high-dose glucocorticoids and cyclophosphamide, with the addition of plasmapheresis in some cases (Goodpasture syndrome, in particular), is the current standard treatment for ANCA-associated vasculitis, Goodpasture syndrome, and SLE presenting with a pulmonary-renal syndrome; this aggressive regimen is warranted even in dialysis-dependent patients, because return of renal function is possible.

- Provide methylprednisolone 500–1000 mg IV once daily × 3–5 days, followed by 1–2 mg/kg daily (IV or po). Alveolar hemorrhage usually stops after 3 to 7 days.

- Cyclophosphamide should be added for better control, faster tapering of steroids, and avoidance of relapses.

  - Many administration protocols are possible: 2 mg/kg IV or orally once a day; or 15 mg/kg IV every 2 weeks × 3 doses, and then every 3 weeks × 6 doses.
  - Pulse or daily administration should be adjusted for renal function.
  - Carefully check for drug-induced neutropenia (often after the seventh day of treatment), and consider lowering cyclophosphamide dose when the WBC count is on a clear downward trend and approaches 4.0×10^{-9}/L.

- Rituximab is an alternative to cyclophosphamide in ANCA-associated vasculitis, particularly in relapsing disease in patients previously exposed to cyclophosphamide.

- Trimethoprim-sulfamethoxazole DS (Septra) 3 times per week (or its equivalent) should be added in all cases to prevent *Pneumocystis jirovecii* infection. Monitoring daily sputum cultures in the ICU patients makes sense. Start early empiric antibiotic therapy in suspected infection.

- Daily plasmapheresis (plasma exchange) should be quickly started in suspected Goodpasture syndrome to remove circulating pathogenic anti-GBM antibodies. Levels of anti-GBM are followed until they normalize, which usually requires about 14 plasmapheresis sessions. Plasmapheresis may be beneficial in ANCA-associated vasculitis with life-threatening disease and in severe kidney disease with dialysis requirement. The role of this therapy continues to be studied.

Further Reading

McCabe C, Jones Q, Nikolopoulou A, et al. Pulmonary-renal syndromes: an update for respiratory physicians. *Respir Med*. 2011;105(10):1413–21. http://dx.doi.org/10.1016/j.rmed.2011.05.012. Medline:21684732

West SC, Arulkumaran N, Ind PW, et al. Pulmonary-renal syndrome: a life threatening but treatable condition. *Postgrad Med J*. 2013;89(1051):274–83. http://dx.doi.org/10.1136/postgradmedj-2012-131416. Medline:23349383

Pul/renal syndrome

16

Scleroderma Renal Crisis

DR. JANET POPE
WESTERN UNIVERSITY, ONTARIO

KEY CONCEPTS

Scleroderma renal crisis (SRC) is characterized by the acute onset of malignant hypertension and progressive renal failure over days to weeks. Elevated blood pressure (new-onset significant hypertension) occurs in 90% of cases, with increased creatinine occurring in 50% of cases at onset and/or microangiopathic hemolytic anemia occurring in 45% of cases.

1. SRC consists of some or all of the following features:

   - elevated creatinine
   - evidence of microangiopathic hemolytic anemia
   - hypertension
   - a clinical picture of systemic sclerosis (SSc/scleroderma) (often the active diffuse SSc subset)

2. It is associated with high plasma renin levels and is analogous to malignant hypertension.

3. SRC may be the first medical presentation or an early presentation of scleroderma, so a high index of suspicion is needed. There is usually a history of recent-onset Raynaud phenomenon and there may be early skin changes such as puffy fingers.

4. Although SRC is rare (3% of scleroderma cases and approximately 15% of the diffuse-subset cases), it can be lethal if not identified and appropriately treated. Treatment involves angiotensin-converting enzyme inhibitors (ACE inhibitors).

5. It is a medical emergency and the more quickly blood pressure (BP) is controlled, the less likely chronic renal failure will result, which can require dialysis or lead to death.

6. ACE inhibitors—the first-line therapy in SRC—have decreased the mortality rate, but the mortality rate is still high.

7. Steroids significantly increase the risk of SRC and should be used only with caution in patients with high risk of developing SRC, such as patients with rapidly progressing skin involvement.

8. Because SRC can be an acute or chronic condition, BP should be watched carefully and monitored as it is in preeclampsia—a small increase in BP should be considered a warning in the early diffuse scleroderma subset. Patients can measure BP daily or every few days in the high-risk group (this group includes patients with the early diffuse subset, especially with tendon friction rubs and increasing or marked skin involvement). The target should be normal BP: a sudden rise in BP (i.e., if BP is usually 120/70 and rises to 180/110) signals the need for immediate medical attention.

9. Since SRC can recur, ACE inhibitors should never be discontinued.

History

PATIENT DEMOGRAPHICS

- Patients with diffuse and progressing scleroderma are at high risk for SRC (high skin score and rapidly progressing skin score). SRC occurs in 3% of SSc patients overall and up to 15% of patients with the early diffuse SSc subset.

- Often patients test positive for RNA polymerase III antibodies—but this is not a routine part of the extractable nuclear antigen (ENA) panel.

- Not all features of SRC need be present. These features include:
  - hypertension
  - rising creatinine
  - anemia with intravascular hemolysis: evidence of schistocytes and other features of RBC breakdown on a peripheral blood smear
- Patients with SRC often have other organ involvement (cardiac, pulmonary, GI). However, SRC may be an initial manifestation of SSc in a patient with new-onset Raynaud phenomenon and puffy fingers, along with a positive antinuclear antibody (ANA) result, before the development of rapidly (often) progressive skin sclerosis with or without tendon friction rubs.
- Glucocorticoid use, especially more than 10 mg prednisone daily, seems to be a risk factor.

KEY QUESTIONS
Note that SRC is **asymptomatic initially**.

1. Is there a history of scleroderma?
- SRC often occurs in the first few years of those with diffuse scleroderma.
- It often occurs with active disease (worsening skin tightening).

2. Are there triggers?
- Ask about steroid use (especially in high dose), because it is an important risk factor.
- Often SRC is exacerbated by other renal insults, such as dehydration (e.g., with diuretic use).

Physical Examination
General appearance: Patients often have diffuse skin changes and look sick.

Vital signs: Patients usually have very elevated BP, both systolic and diastolic (but not necessarily: SRC can occur in the absence of hypertension).

Skin and nails:

- Look for obvious scleroderma with diffuse disease.
- Look for superficial dilated nail fold capillaries.
- Examine for tendon friction rubs (identified by placing the palmar aspect of the fingers across the tendon area being examined and feeling a leathery, rubbing, "squeaking" sensation while the patient moves the underlying joint through its full range of motion).
- Look for puffy fingers (early SSc without other skin involvement).
- Look for telangiectasia especially on hands, face, and mouth.

Cardiovascular exam: Pericardial effusions are common in SRC (echocardiographically), but often not clinically evident.

Respiratory exam: This may detect interstitial lung disease (crackles at bases) associated with scleroderma.

Key Laboratory Investigations

No tests are confirmatory.

INITIAL INVESTIGATIONS

CBC, peripheral smear: Look for microangiopathic hemolytic anemia (fragmented cells, schistocytes, tear drop cells, etc.), consumptive thrombocytopenia.

Creatinine: This is elevated in half of patients.

Urinalysis: This is usually normal, or reveals only mild proteinuria with few cells or casts.

Electrolytes: Potassium should be monitored closely in the context of acute kidney injury.

ANA: This is usually positive, especially in a nucleolar pattern.

ENA: Patients are positive for RNA polymerase III antibody, but this test is often not available as part of the ENA. The presence of RNA polymerase III antibody is associated with a 13-fold increased risk of developing SRC.

ADDITIONAL TESTS

Plasma renin activity: This may be elevated to twice the upper limit of normal or greater. This test is usually not done, because the level may be elevated in active diffuse scleroderma even without SRC.

Lactate dehydrogenase (LD/LDH):

- This is often elevated, but is not specific or sensitive.
- **Note:** LD (LDH) and renin are often elevated in active early diffuse SSc, and so cannot reliably rule SRC in or out.

CK: This may be increased as a result of concomitant:

- scleroderma myopathy or myositis
- cardiac injury due to acute hypertension, often with a slight rise in troponins

Echocardiogram: SRC seems to be associated in some patients with a pericardial effusion. Signs of chronic hypertension such as left ventricular hypertrophy are usually not seen in acute SRC.

Renal biopsy: This is not typically indicated because it does not definitively establish the diagnosis of scleroderma renal disease (it will show thrombotic microangiopathy, which may also be seen in other nonscleroderma causes of this presentation).

Imaging
No imaging is indicated.

Differential Diagnosis
The differential diagnosis includes:

- other causes of hypertension and renal insufficiency (e.g., nonsteroidal anti-inflammatory drugs superimposed on dehydration)
- malignant nephrosclerosis (due to accelerated hypertension), hemolytic-uremic syndrome, thrombotic thrombocytopenic purpura (which may have fever and neurologic phenomena)
- antiphospholipid antibody syndrome (which may have multiple organ involvement with arterial and/or venous thrombi)
- other causes of anemia
  - anemia due to blood loss (common in SSc)
    - erosive esophagitis with bleeding
    - bleeding from telangiectasia with gastric antral vascular ectasia (GAVE) or "watermelon stomach"
    - anemia of chronic disease
  - intravascular hemolysis (**not common** except in SRC)

Initial Therapy
- Ensure the patient's airway, breathing, and circulation (ABCs), including rehydration.
- Ensure rapid control of BP.
  - SRC usually occurs in the setting of a normotensive patient and represents

new severe hypertension. This is unlike hypertensive crisis in someone with preexisting hypertension, where the target BP may be above normal and is achieved more slowly.

- In SRC, monitor BP every 30 minutes to 1 hour, and treat the patient with more doses (oral or IV) of antihypertensives until BP is rapidly normalized.

- Primary drug therapy is with ACE inhibitors (captopril, enalapril best studied). They reduce mortality from 80% to 20%.

- Note that angiotensin II receptor blockers **do not** have same benefit as ACE inhibitors: **ACE inhibitors must be used.**

- Add any antihypertensive to achieve control (such as calcium channel blockers, IV or oral vasodilators). Even alpha blockers, ganglion blockers, or beta blockers can be added in difficult cases.

- Consider dialysis for hyperkalemia, uremia, and fluid overload. If the patient requires dialysis, maintain the ACE inhibitor, because the kidneys may recover even after several months.

- Anemia may need treatment (e.g., blood transfusions).

- Other organ involvement often accompanies SRC: pericardial effusions and other cardiac involvement, interstitial lung disease, pulmonary arterial hypertension, active Raynaud phenomenon, gastroesophageal reflux disease, dysphagia. Specific therapy may be required for these problems.

- Poor outcomes are associated with:
  - longer time to achieve good BP control: modify the antihypertensives every couple of hours

- initial renal insufficiency
- older age

Prophylaxis

- ACE inhibitors **do not** prevent SRC, but prophylactic use may delay the diagnosis and is associated with a worse outcome.
- Patients with early SSc (especially the diffuse subset) should have their BP monitored frequently (e.g., suggest purchase of a BP machine to use at home).
  - A sudden new increase in systolic and diastolic BP should be taken seriously if present on repeated monitoring.
  - Patients often have new-onset acute hypertension symptoms such as headache and blurred vision, but not reliably.

Final Comment

SRC has a poor prognosis and often these patients later die of their overall scleroderma disease burden. Failure to recognize SRC increases the mortality, because an ACE inhibitor **must** be started and used indefinitely (except if relatively contraindicated, such as in future pregnancy when the patient is stable).

Further Reading

Helfrich DJ, Banner B, Steen VD, et al. Normotensive renal failure in systemic sclerosis. *Arthritis Rheum*. 1989;32(9):1128–34. http://dx.doi.org/10.1002/anr.1780320911. Medline:2775321

Muangchan C; Canadian Scleroderma Research Group, Baron M, Pope J. The 15% rule in scleroderma: the frequency of severe organ complications in systemic sclerosis. A systematic review. *J Rheumatol*. 2013;40(9):1545–56. http://dx.doi.org/10.3899/jrheum.121380. Medline:23858045

Seibold JR. Connective tissue diseases characterized by fibrosis. In: Kelley W, Harris E, Ruddy S, et al, editors. Textbook of rheumatology. 5th ed. Philadelphia: W.B. Saunders; 1997. p. 1133–68.

SSc renal crisis

Steen VD. Scleroderma renal crisis. *Rheum Dis Clin North Am*. 2003;29(2):315–33. http://dx.doi.org/10.1016/S0889 -857X(03)00016-4. Medline:12841297

Steen VD, Medsger TA Jr. Case-control study of corticosteroids and other drugs that either precipitate or protect from the development of scleroderma renal crisis. *Arthritis Rheum*. 1998;41(9):1613–9. http://dx.doi.org/10.1002/1529-0131(199809)41:9<1613::AID -ART11>3.0.CO;2-O. Medline:9751093

Steen VD, Medsger TA Jr. Long-term outcomes of scleroderma renal crisis. *Ann Intern Med*. 2000;133(8):600–3. http:// dx.doi.org/10.7326/0003-4819-133-8-200010170-00010. Medline:11033587

Tangri V, Hewson C, Baron M, et al. Associations with organ involvement and autoantibodies in systemic sclerosis: results from the Canadian Scleroderma Research Group (CSRG). *Open J Rheumatol Autoimmune Dis*. 2013;3(02):113–8. http://www.scirp. org/journal/ojra. http://dx.doi.org/10.4236/ojra.2013.32017.

Walker KM, Pope J; participating members of the Scleroderma Clinical Trials Consortium (SCTC); Canadian Scleroderma Research Group (CSRG). Treatment of systemic sclerosis complications: what to use when first-line treatment fails—a consensus of systemic sclerosis experts. *Semin Arthritis Rheum*. 2012;42(1):42–55. http://dx.doi. org/10.1016/j.semarthrit.2012.01.003. Medline:22464314

SECTION 5: APPROACH TO PHYSICAL EXAMINATION IN RHEUMATIC DISEASES

17

The Screening Musculoskeletal Examination

DR. LORI ALBERT
UNIVERSITY OF TORONTO

KEY CONCEPTS

1. Musculoskeletal (MSK) problems are common in inpatient and outpatient settings.
2. Attention to other medical problems may lessen time available for a complete rheumatologic assessment.
3. MSK disorders may affect patient morbidity and mortality, and impair rehabilitation efforts.
4. A screening MSK history and examination will allow the physician to rapidly assess the patient for MSK problems in the context of their other medical issues. It is important to routinely screen for MSK disease on history.
5. A **GALS** (**g**ait, **a**rms, **l**egs, **s**pine) screening examination or other screening examination is easy to incorporate into the physical examination skill set and to use in all patients.

MSK problems are common. While MSK issues may not be the primary or presenting problem for a patient, these issues may influence the patient's ability to rehabilitate from other medical problems, or may interfere with health maintenance by limiting ambulation or other forms of exercise. A screening examination can also enable a rapid assessment of other joints in a patient presenting with monoarthritis.

Several screening examinations have been developed[1-3] including GALS,[1] which is practical and validated.

History

A screening history should be simple and designed to highlight the joint areas of concern, as well as any functional difficulties.

The history portion used in the GALS assessment is brief and includes 3 screening questions:

- Do you have any pain or stiffness in your muscles, joints, or back?
- Can you dress yourself completely without any difficulty?
- Can you walk up and down stairs without any difficulty?

These questions can easily be incorporated into your functional inquiry.

Examination

- There are several different approaches to the screening examination. The basic principle is to do a limited examination of each joint area, using inspection and key manoeuvres that are sensitive to underlying pathological conditions.
- The order in which the joints are examined is not important: the examination should be integrated into the complete physical examination in a rational way.
- Practicing a routine, however, ensures that joints will not be missed.
- In the screening examination, the patient is observed while walking (gait), standing (and/or sitting), and lying down.

- **Standing MSK screen:** This can be done after watching the patient walk and can be integrated with neurologic testing in the lower extremities.
- **Sitting MSK screen:** The cervical spine and upper body MSK screen can be done standing or sitting. If done sitting, it can be easily integrated with vital signs, head and neck examination, and neurologic testing in the upper extremities.
- **Lying MSK screen:** This can be integrated into the supine cardiovascular, abdomen, lymph nodes, and peripheral vascular examinations.

- Ideally, the patient is in underwear, or shorts and a tank top: good visibility is essential for making key observations about deformities, derangements, swelling, discolouration, etc. In addition, symmetry is expected between sides, and the appearance of **asymmetry** may be a clue to an inflamed or damaged joint.

  - Features indicating an **inflamed** joint are swelling, discolouration, warmth, tenderness, and limitation of movement.
  - Features indicating a **damaged** joint are bony enlargement, tenderness, palpable or audible crepitus, and limitation of movement.

GAIT

Observation of gait can be done as the patient enters and exits the room. (Sometimes observing gait after the assessment can serve to corroborate patient history and physical examination findings).

- Gait is ideally observed with the patient in bare feet to assess the phases of gait, as well as alignment and movement at the ankle, midfoot, and MTP joints.
- Ask the patient to put their shoes on and observe the gait again. Check whether footwear compensates for any abnormalities.

- Look for symmetry and smoothness of movement, including: normal stride length; normal phases of gait (heel strike, stance, toe off, and swing through); quick and smooth turning.

WITH PATIENT STANDING OR SITTING

With the patient standing, the spine can be evaluated from behind, from the side, and from the front (cervical). Inspection of the legs is also useful with the patient standing. Examination of the arms, both inspection and movement, can be done in this position if the patient can tolerate standing. Otherwise, this can be done in the sitting position (this may also facilitate integration with other aspects of the physical examination).

From behind the patient:

Examine the spine: Look for evidence of scoliosis (use asymmetry of skin folds or height of pelvic brim or shoulder blades to help you).

Examine the legs: Is there evidence of Baker (popliteal) cyst? How are the knees aligned (varus or valgus)? Is there clear definition of the Achilles tendon? Is there pronation or supination of hind foot?

From the side of the patient:

Examine the spine: Assess for normal cervical and lumbar lordosis and thoracic kyphosis (normally mild).

Assess flexibility of spine and hips: Ask the patient to bend forward and touch their toes.

From the front of the patient:

Examine the spine: The cervical spine can be screened by asking the patient to bend their head sideways to "touch the ear to the shoulder" on each side. The GALS examination uses this movement only for screening the cervical spine.

However, rotation ("look over your shoulder"), and forward flexion or extension ("touch your chin to your chest," "tilt your head to look up at the ceiling"), can also be assessed quickly.

Examine the legs: Is there normal bulk and symmetry in the quadriceps? Is there swelling around the knees or in the suprapatellar pouch? Is there normal alignment of ankle and foot? Are the arches maintained? Is there swelling of the foot or around the ankle? Is there malalignment of toes (claw toes, hammer toes, etc.)?

Examine the arms: In addition to inspection, there are now active movements that need to be done (see the following section).

STEPS IN ARM EXAMINATION

Shoulders

Look for shoulder swelling, muscle wasting.

Assess for normal range of motion. Glenohumeral, sternoclavicular, and acromioclavicular joints are assessed with a single movement—placing the hands behind the head with the elbows pressed back—in the GALS examination. However, individual movements can be quickly assessed:

- The patient starts each movement with the hands in neutral position at the sides.
- Ask the patient to:
  - forward flex the arms until they are beside the ears
  - abduct the arms until they are up beside the ears
  - reach behind the back on each side to touch the inferior tip of the opposite shoulder blade (internal rotation and adduction)
  - place the hands behind the head with elbows pressed back into the coronal plane (external rotation and abduction)

Elbows

Assess elbows by having the patient extend the arms
in front of the body and then flex the elbows to
bring the hands to the shoulders.

Hands and wrists

Look for swelling in the wrists and fingers (e.g.,
fusiform swelling of rheumatoid arthritis, Heberden
and Bouchard nodes of osteoarthritis) or deformities
(e.g., swan neck or boutonniere changes).

Assess:

- Can all the fingers be fully straightened?
- Can a normal fist be made?
- Are there normal "valleys" between MCP joints
  while fingers are in a fist? (Loss of the valleys
  implies swelling at the MCPs.)
- A gentle squeeze across MCPs 2–5 with the hand
  in a neutral position may elicit pain if there is
  synovitis.
- Supination and pronation should be checked for
  range of motion and symmetry.

WITH PATIENT LYING DOWN

Legs

Look for quadriceps muscle wasting, knee swelling,
or asymmetry that was missed when the patient
was standing. Palpate the patella to assess for
subtle warmth that may indicate inflammation.

Assess:

- Use flexion and rotation to assess range of motion
  in the hips and knees. Flexion is active ("bring
  your knee to your chest"). Rotation is passive,
  with hip at 90° and knee at 90°. Rotation is
  sensitive to hip joint disease.
- Knee flexion can be done actively and/or passively
  while evaluating range of motion in the hips.

Screening exam

Feet

Look for calluses on the soles of the feet that can indicate uneven pressure due to lower extremity joint problems.

Assess: Squeeze the MTP joints gently to screen for synovitis.

Recording the Findings of the Screening Examination

- You should record a normal screening examination for future reference.

- If an abnormality in a joint is suspected from the screen, it should be recorded, but that joint should also be examined in more detail by using the techniques described in chapter 18.

- Table 17.1 shows an example record of a normal GALS screening examination. Table 17.2 shows an example record of a "positive" screening examination.

TABLE 17.1. Example of normal screening examination recorded as in the GALS assessment[1]

Gait	✓	Appearance	Movement
Arms		✓	✓
Legs		✓	✓
Spine		✓	✓

TABLE 17.2. Example of an abnormal screening examination recorded as in the GALS assessment

Gait	✓	Appearance	Movement
Arms		✓	X*
Legs		✓	✓
Spine		X**	✓

*Limitation of left shoulder range of motion.

**Accentuated thoracic kyphosis.

- Keep track of any abnormalities detected on your examination to see if a pattern emerges that may be helpful in establishing a diagnosis.

References

1. Doherty M, Dacre J, Dieppe P, et al. The 'GALS' locomotor screen. *Ann Rheum Dis*. 1992;51(10):1165–9. http://dx.doi.org/10.1136/ard.51.10.1165. Medline:1444632

2. Coady D, Walker D, Kay L. Regional Examination of the Musculoskeletal System (REMS): a core set of clinical skills for medical students. *Rheumatology (Oxford)*. 2004;43(5):633–9. http://dx.doi.org/10.1093/rheumatology/keh138. Medline:15054154

3. Thompson JM. The musculoskeletal screening examination [Internet]. Canadian Rheumatology Association; 1998. [cited 2014 Oct 4]. Available from: http://rheum.ca/images/documents/The_Musculoskeletal_Screening_Examination_Booklet.pdf

Further Resources

Cividino A, Miettunen P, Haraoui B. [Video series], GALS exam [Internet]. Canadian Rheumatology Association; c2014; 2011. [cited 2014 Oct 4]. Available from: http://rheum.ca/en/students/student_educational_resources

18

The Detailed Joint Examination

DR. EVELYN SUTTON
DALHOUSIE UNIVERSITY

This chapter provides a framework for a detailed joint examination when a screening examination suggests specific joint abnormalities.

KEY CONCEPTS

1. You need to remember basic functional anatomy.
2. Approach each joint in an organized fashion and test hypotheses as you go.
3. Your goal on examination is to be able to determine whether a joint is normal or abnormal.
4. If it is abnormal, is it **inflammatory** or **degenerative** joint disease?
5. Joint swelling should be identified as arising from increased intra-articular fluid, hypertrophied synovium (both inflammatory), or bony enlargement (degenerative).
6. If you determine that a patient has joint disease, the pattern of joint involvement, the nature of swelling (bony or fluid), and the duration of symptoms will aid in formulating a specific diagnosis.
7. Detailed joint examinations are an important part of monitoring patients with chronic inflammatory arthritis. A joint count can provide a record of disease activity and change over time.

Basic Principles

If a joint is swollen because of increased fluid:

- It is **most likely sore**. The body will consciously or unconsciously try to protect it. The normal movement (range of motion) will be decreased in at least 2 planes, usually flexion and extension.

- It is **warm to the touch**.

- The **patient protects it**, both consciously and unconsciously. A sore, weight-bearing joint will result in an antalgic (pain-relieving) gait; a sore upper limb joint will be held close to the body to protect it.

- It is **possibly red**. Erythema is an important sign and indicates inflammation. Characteristically gouty joints are brighter and hotter than rheumatoid joints and even septic joints. If there is desquamation about the joint, gout is nearly always the cause.

Examine all joints using the same approach: **inspection, palpation, range of motion, special tests**.

INSPECTION

- Always compare 1 part with its counterpart simultaneously.

- Make sure you get more than 1 view; for the hands and wrists, inspect the radial, ulnar, palmar, and dorsal planes.

- Examine elbows, shoulders, hips, knees, and ankles. Make sure to look anteriorly, posteriorly, and laterally.

- In the feet, do not use only a "bird's-eye view" (i.e., the top of the foot); also get a "worm's-eye view" (i.e., the sole of the foot).

- Look for alignment, bony and/or soft tissue swelling, erythema, nodules, skin changes, and periarticular muscle atrophy around all joints.

Joint exam

PALPATION

- Palpate each joint to identify tenderness, effusions, bony enlargement, and crepitus.
- Identify the important bony and soft tissue landmarks for each major joint.
  - The bony landmarks are particularly important in the evaluation of the swollen joint, as they form the reference points needed for proper joint aspiration and/or injection.
- Assess heat in the wrists, elbows, knees, and ankles.
  - Do not waste your time trying to assess heat in the shoulder or hip joints; they are covered by muscle that, by nature, is metabolically active and hence, should be warm.
  - Knees, elbows, and ankles are close to the surface and should be cooler than muscle.
  - Fingers and toes are usually at ambient temperature and temperature evaluation is unreliable.
- Feel for a joint effusion. Evaluate the bursae for swelling. They will feel fluid-filled when swollen. Bony enlargement will be hard, with no fluctuance.
- Palpate the joint line and tendon insertions for tenderness.
- Palpate for crepitus during range of motion.

RANGE OF MOTION

- Active range of motion should be done first.
- When active range of motion is unrestricted and without protected movements, no assessment of passive range of motion is needed.
- When active range is restricted, passive range must be assessed.
- Examination of the hip is unique: it usually skips active range and proceeds directly to passive range of motion.

SPECIAL TESTS
Tendon inflammation or damage
- Regardless of their name, these tests all use the same principle of stretch and stress.
- If you can vaguely remember where a tendon attaches, you can assess it by putting it under a stretch or a stress.
- The stretch can be passive or active. If a tendon is inflamed, stretching it will cause pain.
- Since other structures are also stretched (e.g., skin, superficial nerves), you can test the same tendon by putting it under stress (i.e., resisting muscle-powered movement of the tendon).

Ligamentous integrity
- These tests are based solely on applying a stretching force across the ligament, and evaluating joint movement and patient report of pain.
- A minimum number of named tests are included in this chapter, but they are so well-known that it is important to be familiar with them.

Joint count or articular index
- This is a summation of the number of "active" joints (inflamed joints) to assist the clinician in monitoring the effectiveness of therapy.
- Several different articular indexes for disease activity exist (see references) which are used routinely in clinical practice to determine disease activity and inform therapeutic decisions.
- The number of swollen joints and the number of tender joints are important components in most of these validated indexes.
- You should be able to evaluate a patient for clinically active joints and to summarize with an active joint count.

Joint-count diagrams

You should try to record your joint examination with a diagram.

- A diagram gives a complete and easy-to-read representation of the involved joints, and a diagnostic pattern may become evident. It is also easy to follow clinical improvement if each evaluation is noted in this way.

- You should define a legend for your diagram, for example:

  X = tender joint

  ● = effused joint

- Note specific deformities on the diagram. For example, the patient in Figure 18.1 has 38 swollen joints, in a pattern suggestive of RA—small and large joints, symmetrically distributed in both lower and upper extremities.

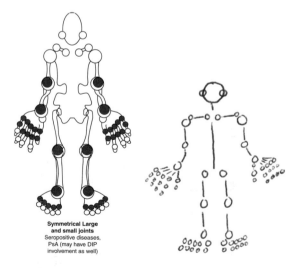

Symmetrical Large and small joints
Seropositive diseases, PsA (may have DIP involvement as well)

FIGURE 18.1. Diagrams are a way to record joint counts. You can easily learn to draw your own homunculus with practice.

Specific Joint Examination

It is not possible to itemize all the aspects of the musculoskeletal examination in this text, but a quick summary of key examination points for each region is given here.

HAND EXAMINATION

Inspection

- Look for normal alignment of the fingers and record any abnormalities.
- Bony enlargement of the DIP and PIP joints is classic for osteoarthritis and can be recognized immediately (Figures 18.2 and 18.3).
- Swan neck and boutonniere deformities (Figures 18.4 and 18.5) are seen in inflammatory arthritides.
- Mallet finger deformities (Figure 18.6) can result from trauma or from inflammatory arthritis.
- The presence of nail pits is strongly associated with psoriatic arthritis.

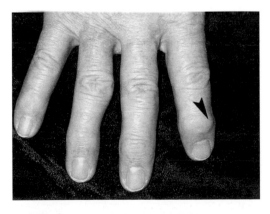

FIGURE 18.2. Heberden node on right second DIP joint.

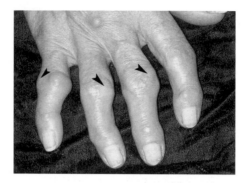

FIGURE 18.3. Bouchard nodes on PIP joints of right hand.

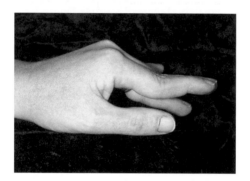

FIGURE 18.4. Swan neck deformity of left index finger.

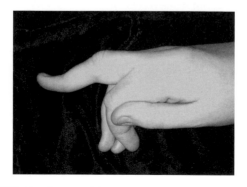

FIGURE 18.5. Boutonniere deformity of right third digit.

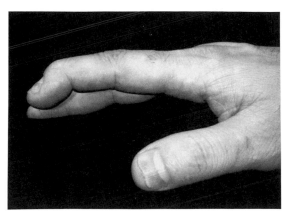

FIGURE 18.6. Mallet finger deformity of right second digit.

Palpation

Be comfortable with the 4-finger technique for finger joint evaluation (Figure 18.7).

- If the joint is enlarged, palpation should confirm whether the enlargement is from:
  - new bone formation: feels like the bridge of your nose (same texture and feel)
  - excess fluid in the joint: feels like squeezing a grape (the 4-finger technique provides maximum sensitivity)
  - thickening of the synovium (from hypertrophy, hyperplasia, or tumour of synovium): feels like pressing your finger against your cheekbone (soft, but hard underneath)
- Check the palm for thickening of the palmar fascia by running your thumb across the patient's palm.

Range of motion

Normal fingers can tuck fully into the palm, with all finger pads in contact with the palmar surface of the corresponding MCP joint. They can also

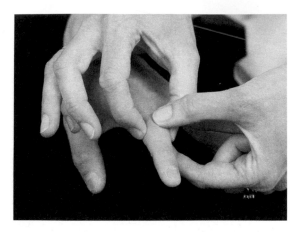

FIGURE 18.7. Four-finger technique for PIP joint evaluation.

make a fist, which requires full flexion of the MCP joints.

- If there is no restriction in doing either of these 2 manoeuvres, there is no significant abnormality in the DIP, PIP, or MCP joints.
- If the patient is unable to do these manoeuvres, you must assess passive range of motion of the affected fingers.

WRIST EXAMINATION

Inspection

Examine ulnar, radial, palmar, and dorsal views. Look for swelling, erythema, and/or deformity.

- Swelling over the radial aspect of the joint is nearly always due to osteoarthritic change in the thumb carpal-metacarpal joint, or from tenosynovitis of the extensor pollicis brevis and abductor pollicis longus tendons (De Quervain tendons).
- Swelling over the ulnar aspect of the wrist in the absence of trauma is specific for inflammatory joint disease.

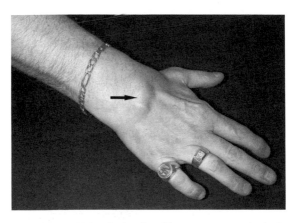

FIGURE 18.8. "Tuck sign" with swelling of the common extensor tendon sheath.

- The common extensor tendon sheath of the second to the fifth fingers is frequently swollen in rheumatoid arthritis; with finger extension, the synovium buckles and the "tuck sign" is apparent (Figure 18.8).

Palpation
- Check for increased heat, making sure to compare to muscle, not tendon.
- Identify the ulnar styloid, radial tubercle, scaphoid, and pisiform.
- At the base of the second and third metacarpals and just distal to the radial tubercle, there is normally an indentation where the proximal carpal row is easily palpable. If the wrist is swollen, fullness will be evident in this region.

Range of motion
Flexion, extension, radial and ulnar deviation, pronation, and supination should be checked. The elbow must be held in 90° flexion to eliminate humeral contribution.

Special tests

The Phalen (Figure 18.9), Tinel (Figure 18.10), and Finkelstein tests are well described in all the standard textbooks and should be reviewed and learned.

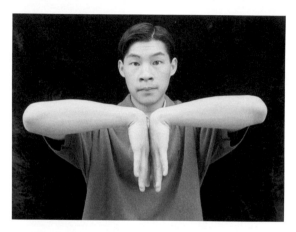

FIGURE 18.9. The Phalen test.

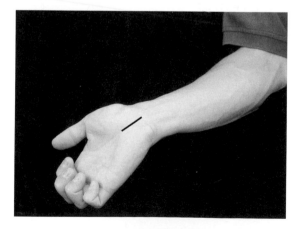

FIGURE 18.10. The Tinel test: the black line shows the location for percussion over the median nerve.

ELBOW EXAMINATION

Inspection

The patient should be standing, if possible, for this part of the examination. Note the carrying angle, as well as the presence of any nodules and bursal swelling.

Palpation

- Check for heat over the extensor surface of the joint.
- Identify the bony landmarks: medial and lateral epicondyles, radial head, and olecranon.
- Palpate the olecranon bursa for swelling and the presence of nodules.
- Assess the joint for effusion; the normal recesses between the olecranon and epicondyles are lost when excess fluid is present in the joint.

Range of motion

- Check flexion, extension, pronation, and supination.
- Remember to assess pronation and supination with the elbow at 90° flexion.

Special tests

Use the principle of stretch and stress to test for medial and lateral epicondylitis (golfer's and tennis elbow, respectively).

- Resisted extension of the wrist produces pain from lateral epicondylitis.
- Resisted palmar flexion of the wrist produces pain from medial epicondylitis.

SHOULDER EXAMINATION

The shoulder examination involves 3 synovial joints (sternoclavicular, acromioclavicular, and glenohumeral) and 1 articulation (scapulothoracic).

The complete shoulder examination requires evaluation of all components.

Inspection

Compare both shoulders. Swelling of the shoulders may be subtle, with loss of the pectoral-deltoid groove the only visible sign. Large joint effusions may cause the shoulder to look globally enlarged.

Palpation

- Ask the patient where the shoulder hurts and palpate this area last.
- Identify the spine of the scapula, the posterior and anterior edges of the acromion, the acromioclavicular joint, and the sternoclavicular joint.
- Check for tenderness at the insertion of the rotator cuff tendons; identify the bicipital groove and the long head of the biceps.

Range of motion

Full active unrestricted and unprotected movement of the shoulders effectively rules out significant pathology in the shoulder joints and no more testing is required in that instance.

- Ask the patient to bring their hands behind their head, and then down behind their back, forward and up over their head, and then slowly down to their sides.
- If there is hesitation or restriction of any movements, do them passively.
- Look for early scapulothoracic movement (i.e., shrugging of the shoulder with abduction and flexion); this is a sign of glenohumeral disease.

Special tests

The principle of putting tendons under stretch and stress is put to excellent use in the shoulder examination.

- Stretch the bicipital tendons by extending the shoulder and elbow, flexing the wrist, and pronating the forearm. Stress the bicipital tendon by resisting its primary movements (i.e., shoulder and elbow flexion, wrist supination).

- Test the rotator cuff tendons by resisting shoulder external and internal rotation and abduction.

- The supraspinatus can be simultaneously stretched and stressed by resisting upward movement of the internally rotated, abducted, and forward flexed shoulder (Figure 18.11).

- The acromioclavicular joint can be palpated for tenderness and stressed by adducting the flexed shoulder and elbow across the chest (Figure 18.12).

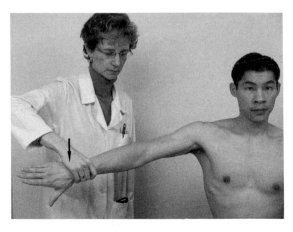

FIGURE 18.11. Stressing the supraspinatus tendon.

Joint exam

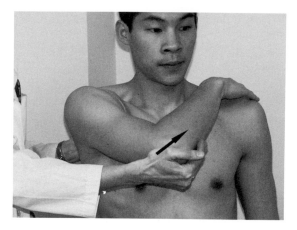

FIGURE 18.12. Stressing the acromioclavicular joint.

CERVICAL SPINE

Inspection
Observe the position of the head relative to the neck and torso.

- Is it held chin forward?
- Is there marked upper thoracic kyphosis affecting the head and neck position?

Palpation
In the screening examination, this can be skipped.

Range of motion
Observe the following motions in the patient: chin up, chin down, looking to the left and right, ear to shoulder. If there is restriction, assess passive range with the patient supine and with gentle movements to see if range can be increased.

Special tests
Deep tendon reflexes of the upper and lower extremity and the Babinski test should be included in the screening rheumatologic examination.

THORACIC SPINE

Inspection
Note the shape of the chest and deformities if present.

Palpation
As in the cervical spine examination, this can be excluded in the screening examination.

Range of motion
This is not required in the screening examination.

Special tests
In patients with suspected or confirmed spondylarthritis, measure chest expansion. Use a tape measure at the nipple line, and measure from end expiration to maximum inspiration. Normal chest expansion is 5 cm.

LUMBAR SPINE AND SI JOINTS
(SEE ALSO CHAPTER 8)

Inspection
- Look for presence or absence of lumbar lordosis, café au lait spots, and patches of hair.
- Identify the dimples of Venus and draw an imaginary line between them to get an idea about leg length discrepancy or pelvic obliquity from scoliosis.

Palpation
- Skip this step in the screening examination.
- To assess a patient with back pain, ask the patient to lie prone. Palpate for tenderness of the muscles, spinous processes, and SI joints. Use common sense: this would not be done in someone suspected of having a fracture.

Range of motion
- Flexion, extension, and side flexion can be done with the patient standing (see details in chapter 8).

- Observe thoracolumbar rotation with the patient sitting so as to fix the pelvis.

Special tests
- You should be comfortable with these: the Schober test (Figure 18.13), the Trendelenburg test (Figure 18.14), and the FABER test (Figure 18.15). These are not expected on a screening examination, but should be included in the workup of a patient suspected of having a spondylarthritis.
- Complete the lumbar spine and SI joint examination with straight leg raising, both sitting and lying, and deep tendon reflexes of the lower extremity (see details in chapter 8).

HIPS

Inspection
Look for abnormal gait pattern (e.g., limp, trunk shift, or lurch) and decreased stance time in 1 or both legs.

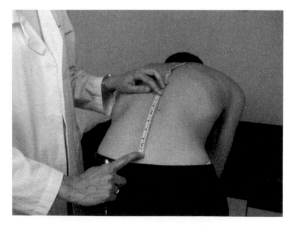

FIGURE 18.13. Position of tape measure for Schober test.

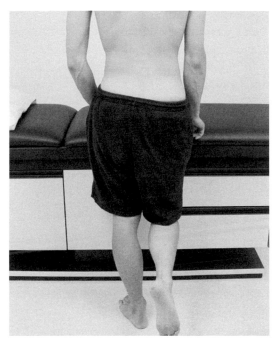

FIGURE 18.14. Positive Trendelenburg test, left hip.

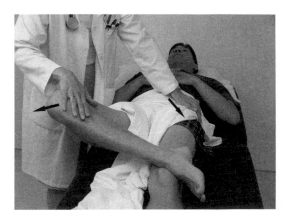

FIGURE 18.15. FABER test: assessing right hip and SI joint.

Palpation

- This is not necessary in a screening examination.
- In a patient with hip region pain, palpate the greater trochanter, anterior and posterior iliac crests, and spines.

Range of motion

Check internal and external rotation, abduction, adduction, flexion, and extension. If the movements produce pain, make note of its location.

- Groin pain is in keeping with hip joint pain.
- Pain over the side of the hip or buttocks is more in keeping with pain from the lumbar spine, SI joints, or trochanteric bursa.

Special tests

- The Trendelenburg and FABER tests should be done as in the "Lumbar Spine and SI Joints" section.
- To test for hip flexion contracture, observe the position of the hip when lumbar lordosis is eliminated (Thomas test, Figure 18.16).

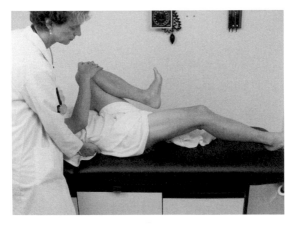

FIGURE 18.16. Thomas test: evidence of flexion contracture in the right hip.

KNEES

Inspection

- Ask the patient to stand and check for varus and valgus deformities, flexion contractures, and "sway back knees" (genu recurvatum).
- Observe gait.

Palpation

- Check for heat, swelling, tenderness, and crepitus.
- Identify the joint line, patella, and bursae.

Range of motion

- Flexion and extension are the primary movements of the knee.
- Tibial inversion and eversion should be assessed in the flexed knee.

Special tests

- Look for small effusions by checking for the bulge sign (Figure 18.17). Large effusions are balloted.
- Test for ligamentous integrity by applying a stretching force to the 4 main ligaments in turn:
  - valgus force for the medial collateral ligament (Figure 18.18)

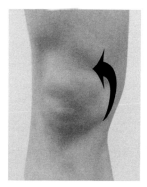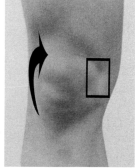

FIGURE 18.17. Bulge test for knee effusion.

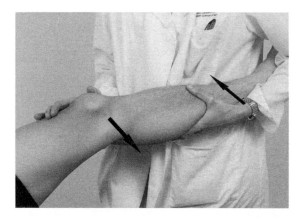

FIGURE 18.18. Applying valgus force to stretch the medial collateral ligament

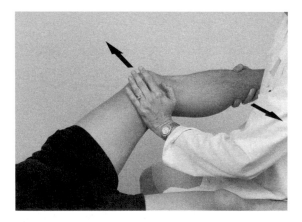

FIGURE 18.19. Applying varus force to stretch the lateral collateral ligament.

- varus force for the lateral collateral ligament (Figure 18.19)
- pulling force for the anterior cruciate ligament (Figure 18.20)
- pushing force for the posterior cruciate ligament (also Figure 18.20)

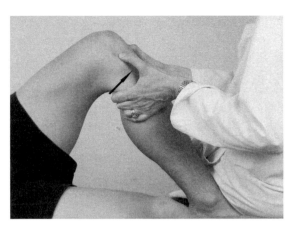

FIGURE 18.20. Testing the anterior cruciate ligament.

- Meniscal integrity should be assessed if a partial or complete tear is suspected by a history of intermittent locking of the knee. The most sensitive test is the Thessaly test and it is the preferred test in patients who do not have a torn anterior cruciate ligament and who can balance standing on 1 leg. The examiner holds the patient's extended hands for balance, asks the patient to stand on 1 leg with the weight-bearing knee flexed to 20°, and then to twist their upper body in 1 direction and then the other 3 times. A positive test exacerbates the pain in the weight-bearing knee. There may be a locking or catching sensation.

ANKLE AND FOOT
Inspection
As with the other weight-bearing joints, initial inspection should be with the patient standing.

- Look for signs of pain on walking with heel strike, plantar flexion, and toe off.

- The medial malleolus should be higher than the lateral malleolus.
- Inspect the Achilles tendon for integrity, nodule formation, and alignment.
- Note alignment abnormalities of the forefoot and for preservation of the longitudinal arch.
- Look for splaying of the toes, a sign of MTP joint swelling.
- Examine the sole of the foot.

Palpation

Evaluate the ankle and foot much as you would the wrist and hand.

- Identify the important bony landmarks: medial and lateral malleoli, navicular, talus, calcaneus, base of the fifth metatarsal, and MTP joints.
- Check for tenderness, warmth, and swelling in the ankles, midfeet, and MTP and interphalangeal joints of the toes.

Range of motion

- The true ankle joint has only 2 movements: dorsi and plantar flexion. This is best observed with the knee flexed so as to relax the gastrocnemius muscles.
- Next, check inversion and eversion of the mid- and forefoot. If active range is restricted, assess passive movement.
- Next, assess toe movement of flexion, extension, abduction, and adduction, keeping in mind the tremendous genetic variability in toe abduction and adduction.
- The subtalar joint can be assessed only by passive range of motion: grasp the calcaneus by cupping the heel, lock the tibiotalar joint in dorsiflexion, and apply varus and valgus forces. Normally, there should be little movement with this manoeuvre.

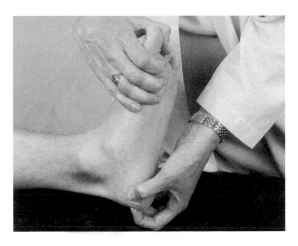

FIGURE 18.21. Applying stretch to the plantar fascia.

Special tests

Plantar fasciitis is common in the spondyloarthritides and should be checked in patients with reports of heel and foot pain.

- Grasp the heel and apply firm pressure to the distal/medial aspect of the calcaneus to see if pain is elicited.
- Stretch the plantar fascia by forcibly extending the toes (Figure 18.21).

Further Reading

Anderson J, Caplan L, Yazdany J, et al. Rheumatoid arthritis disease activity measures: American College of Rheumatology recommendations for use in clinical practice. *Arthritis Care Res (Hoboken)*. 2012;64(5):640–7. http://dx.doi.org/10.1002/acr.21649. Medline:22473918

Karachalios T, Hantes M, Zibis AH, et al. Diagnostic accuracy of a new clinical test (the Thessaly test) for early detection of meniscal tears. *J Bone Joint Surg Am*. 2005;87(5):955–62. http://dx.doi.org/10.2106/JBJS.D.02338. Medline:15866956

SECTION 6: JOINT ASPIRATION AND INJECTION TECHNIQUES

19

Approach to Joint Aspiration and Injection

DR. DENIS CHOQUETTE
UNIVERSITY OF MONTREAL

DR. LORI ALBERT
UNIVERSITY OF TORONTO

Indications for Aspiration of Joints and Injection

DIAGNOSTIC

Aspiration is:

- mandatory if septic arthritis is suspected
  - Serial aspirations may be required to determine response to therapy.
- advised if crystal arthritis or hemarthrosis suspected
- used to clarify diagnosis of arthritis as inflammatory versus noninflammatory

THERAPEUTIC

Aspiration is used for:

- draining tense effusion to relieve pain and reduce intra-articular pressure
- draining blood and purulent joint effusions

Injections involve:

- injection of glucocorticoid for management of a noninfectious inflammatory articular or periarticular process
- injection of viscosupplementation agents (occasionally in combination with glucocorticoid) for management of osteoarthritis

Contraindications to Aspiration of a Joint

ABSOLUTE
Never aspirate a joint with suspected infection, or an open lesion on overlying skin or soft tissues.

RELATIVE
Use caution in the following settings:

- bleeding diathesis
- thrombocytopenia
- prosthetic joint

Contraindications to Injection of a Joint

ABSOLUTE
Never inject a joint in the following settings:

- suspected infection of joint
- bacteremia
- prosthetic joint

RELATIVE
Use injections cautiously in the following settings:

- bleeding diathesis
- thrombocytopenia
- failure to respond to previous injections

Joint injection

Risks

Risks include:

- hemorrhage into joint space
- joint injury
  - This may be avoided by advancing the needle slowly and preventing excessive movement of the needle while in the joint space.
- iatrogenic septic arthritis (*rare:* fewer than 1:10,000 cases)
- tendon rupture (if steroid injected directly into tendon)
  - If resistance to injection is felt, repositioning the needle should help.
- subcutaneous fat atrophy and depigmentation of skin overlying injection site
- cartilage injury with repeated injection (limit injections to 3–4/joint/year)

Procedure

1. GATHER MATERIALS REQUIRED

Full sterile set up is not required as long as the operator is comfortable and the skin around the injection site will not be touched.

Skin preparation

- proviodine solution
- alcohol swabs
- sterile gauze pads
- local anesthetic (1% lidocaine)
- sterile gloves
- adhesive bandage

Syringes and needle

- 21/22-gauge bore needle for nonseptic aspiration (may require 18-gauge for septic fluid)
- 3- to 5-mL syringes for diagnostic purposes (may use larger syringes for therapeutic drainage)

Specimen collection

- sterile specimen container or tube (without anticoagulant) for culture
- tube with anticoagulant for cell count

Lidocaine

- Use lidocaine as indicated, for anaesthetizing skin, soft tissue, and joint to increase comfort during the procedure.
- Note that lidocaine may be mixed with glucocorticoid to ensure good placement and provide immediate relief from pain.

Glucocorticoid preparation (see also chapter 12)

- if therapeutic injection is to be done

2. LANDMARK

- This is critical to a successful procedure (see figures that follow).
- Mark the entry point with a pen (may be erased by cleaning skin) or by creating an indentation in the skin with the tip of the needle cap, closed retractable pen, fingernail, etc.

3. STERILIZE FIELD

- Sterilize the field using 3 concentric outward spirals with iodine disinfectant. Betadine-soaked gauze may be used; ensure nonsterile gloves do not touch the field, or use sterile gloves. Chlorhexidine swabs may also be used. Allow the field to dry.
- Use alcohol (can use swabs, ensuring that nonsterile gloves do not touch the field) to remove Betadine from needle entry point outwards.
- You may check your landmark at this point if you are wearing sterile gloves. Otherwise, a fresh alcohol swab may be placed over the entry site and the nonsterile gloved finger can palpate through the swab to check the landmark (the swab is removed prior to beginning the procedure).

Joint injection

4. PROCEED WITH ASPIRATION/INJECTION (SEE FIGURES THAT FOLLOW)

- Local anaesthetic may be used, but should be avoided if you are aspirating fluid for culture, because it could interfere with the culture.

- Puncture the skin quickly and then proceed more slowly toward the joint space, aspirating as you go. As soon as synovial fluid is obtained, avoid further forward movement of the needle to prevent damage to the cartilage. If resistance is encountered, reposition the needle.

- If fluid is obtained initially and then flow stops:
  - Ensure that surrounding musculature is relaxed (especially for knee aspirations).
  - Reposition the needle in small increments— release the suction initially (synovium may have been drawn up against the bevel of the needle), reposition gently, and then attempt to aspirate again. Gentle rotation of the needle can also help.
  - Reinject some of the fluid in the syringe to relieve a potential blockage in the needle.
  - Apply counter pressure from another area of the joint to "push" fluid toward the needle.

- Once the syringe is full, disconnect it from the hub of the needle and expel the contents of this first aspirate into the sterile specimen container for culture, being careful not to touch the syringe to the sterile container. Reattach this syringe (as long as it is uncontaminated) or attach a fresh syringe for further aspiration.

- Placing a small sterile gauze over the barrel of the needle will improve your grip on the barrel and assist in detaching the syringe. This also keeps the exposed part of the needle sterile in case you have to advance the needle later on (some people also use a small hemostat or clamp). Do this part of the procedure slowly and carefully to avoid inadvertently repositioning the needle, which may cause pain or cause synovial fluid flow to stop.

- Aspirate as much fluid as possible without causing the patient discomfort or repeated repositioning of the needle.
- If a glucocorticoid is to be injected, attach the syringe containing the steroid preparation to the barrel of the needle. Aspirate again to ensure that there is free flow of synovial fluid into the syringe (i.e., the needle is still in the synovial space) before proceeding with injection. There should be minimal resistance to injection of the steroid.
- **Glucocorticoid injection should only be attempted if:**
  - There is no doubt that the needle is in the joint space.
  - Infection has been ruled out.
  - You first aspirate to ensure the needle tip is not in a blood vessel.
  - There is minimal resistance to flow upon injecting.

5. POSTINJECTION CARE

- Apply pressure to the site for a few minutes with clean gauze.
- Keep the injection site clean and dry for 24 hours (to avoid introduction of bacteria).
- Ideally, rest the injected joint for 24 to 48 hours.
- Ice packs 3 to 4 times in the following 24 hours, acetaminophen, nonsteroidal anti-inflammatory drugs may relieve local pain.
- Warn the patient about **postinjection flare**:
  - The patient may experience increased pain/ burning in the joint beginning several hours after the injection. This is thought to be due to

Joint injection

crystallization of the steroid preparation in the joint with secondary inflammation.

- It may last for 1 to 2 days and is self-limited.
- It can be treated with local application of cold and with oral acetaminophen.
- Any postinjection flare that persists or starts late requires attention.

Specific Joint Injections

Specific joint injections are best learned by observation of an experienced operator doing the procedure, followed by performing the technique yourself under supervision.

This section provides figures and descriptions to assist you in learning these procedures.

KNEE ASPIRATION AND INJECTION

The knee is among the simplest joints to access. There are several possible approaches. The medial and lateral approaches are most commonly used. In these approaches:

- The knee is kept extended: a small pillow can be placed under the joint if it enhances palpation of the joint space.

- The needle is inserted about one-third of the way down from the superior pole of the patella, with the needle perpendicular to the skin but directed slightly posteriorly, as the patellar undersurface slopes posteriorly.

- The knee joint can be approached from the medial or lateral aspect of the joint (see Figure 19.1 for medial approach). You should be able to palpate the space with your finger when landmarking. Note that there is greater muscle bulk on the medial aspect but the joint capsule is tougher laterally.

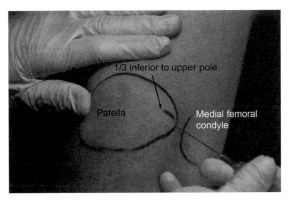

FIGURE 19.1. Medial approach to knee injection and aspiration.

SHOULDER ASPIRATION AND INJECTION

There are several approaches to shoulder injection and aspiration. Glenohumeral joint aspiration may be difficult. If fluid cannot be obtained in the setting of an acute shoulder monoarthritis, fluoroscopic- or ultrasound-guided aspiration is indicated.

Posterior approach

This approach is best for injecting the shoulder.

- The patient is sitting.
- Palpate the posterior margin of the acromion and locate the most posterior and lateral point (the posterior "corner").
- Insert the needle 1 cm below and 1 cm medial to this point, aiming slightly medially toward the coracoid process. The needle should be inserted almost to the hub. There should be no resistance to injection. (See Figure 19.2.)

Anterior approach

This approach is suitable for aspirating a visible shoulder effusion.

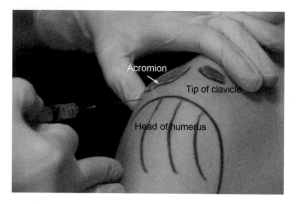

FIGURE 19.2. Posterior approach to should injections.

- The patient is sitting. The arm should hang at the side with the elbow flexed to 90°.
- Palpate the coracoid process and insert the needle 1 cm lateral and 1 cm distal to this point.
- The needle can be directed in a slightly upward direction. This approach is associated with a higher risk of vasovagal syndrome. Do not insert the needle medial to the coracoid process, as this may bring the needle into contact with neurovascular structures.

Subacromial bursa injection

This is used in the setting of subacromial impingement and some cases of calcific tendinitis. In this setting, injection of a mixture of lidocaine and glucocorticoid is used, as relief of pain confirms the diagnosis.

- The patient is sitting. It is helpful to have adequate muscle relaxation to palpate the gap between the acromion and the humeral head.
- Insert the needle laterally under the acromion, aiming slightly anteromedially. There should be easy flow of the mixture.

ANKLE ASPIRATION AND INJECTION

- Injection or aspiration of the tibiotalar joint is accomplished with the patient in the supine position and the foot at a 90° angle with the leg. Some plantar flexion may be helpful in opening the joint.

- Locate the space between the tibia and talus by gently flexing and extending the foot.

- Insert the needle vertically into the joint space bordered by the tibialis anterior tendon laterally and the medial malleolus medially (see Figures 19.3 and 19.4). The needle may be directed slightly toward the lateral malleolus.

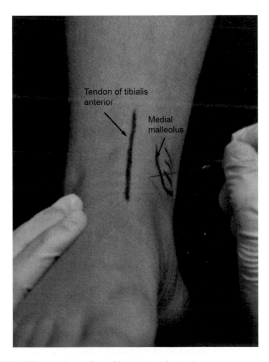

Tendon of tibialis anterior

Medial malleolus

FIGURE 19.3. Approach to ankle injection and aspiration.

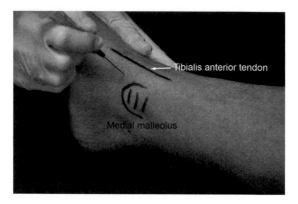

FIGURE 19.4. Approach to ankle injection and aspiration.

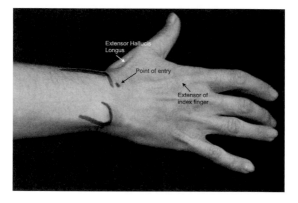

FIGURE 19.5. Surface anatomy relevant to wrist injection and aspiration.

WRIST ASPIRATION AND INJECTION

- The radiocarpal joint can be palpated by gently flexing and extending the wrist. The injection should be done with the wrist relaxed and partially flexed.
- The site for injection is at the distal radius in the small depression between the scaphoid and lunate (see Figures 19.5 and 19.6). Another way

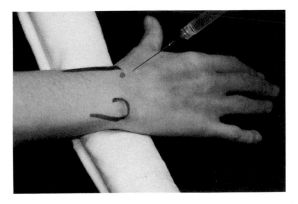

FIGURE 19.6. Injection of the radiocarpal joint.

to localize this space is to follow the thumb and index finger extensor tendons proximally and locate the depression between these tendons at the distal radius.

- The needle should be inserted perpendicular to the skin and may be directed slightly toward the thumb.

Further Reading

Conway R, O'Shea FD, Cunnane G, et al. Safety of joint and soft tissue injections in patients on warfarin anticoagulation. *Clin Rheumatol.* 2013;32(12):1811–4. http://dx.doi.org/10.1007/s10067-013-2350-z. Medline:23925554

Abbreviations

AAV	antineutrophil cytoplasmic antibody (ANCA)-associated vasculitides
ABCDES	alignment, bone, cartilage, distribution, erosions, soft tissue
ABCs	airway, breathing, circulation (with respect to resuscitation)
AC	acromioclavicular
ACE	angiotensin-converting enzyme
aCL	anti-cardiolipin
ACPA	anti-citrullinated protein antibody
ACTH	adrenocorticotropic hormone
AI	aortic insufficiency
AIDS	acquired immunodeficiency syndrome
AKI	acute kidney injury
ALT	alanine aminotransferase
ANA	antinuclear antibody
ANCA	antineutrophil cytoplasmic antibody
anti-CCP	anti-cyclic citrullinated peptide
anti-dsDNA	anti-double-stranded DNA
anti-GBM	anti-glomerular basement membrane
anti-MPO	antimyeloperoxidase
anti-PR3	anti-proteinase 3
anti-β2GPI	antibodies against β2 glycoprotein-I
AP	anteroposterior
aPL	antiphospholipid
APS	antiphospholipid syndrome
aPTT	activated partial thromboplastin time
AS	ankylosing spondylitis
ASA	acetylsalicylic acid
ASAS	Assessment of Spondylarthritis International Society
AST	aspartate aminotransferase
BD	Behçet disease
bid	twice a day
BP	blood pressure
BUN	serum urea nitrogen
C3	complement component 3
C4	complement component 4
cANCA	cytoplasmic antineutrophil cytoplasmic antibody
CBC	complete blood cell count
CCB	calcium channel blocker
CCP	cyclic citrullinated peptide
CK	creatine kinase
CKD/MBD	chronic kidney disease-mineral and bone-related disorders
CMC	carpometacarpal
CNS	central nervous system
COX	cyclo-oxygenase enzyme
CPPD	calcium pyrophosphate dihydrate

CREST	calcinosis, *Raynaud* phenomenon, *e*sophageal motility disorders, *s*clerodactyly, and *t*elangiectasia
CRP	C-reactive protein
CSF	cerebrospinal fluid
CT	computed tomography
CTA	computed tomography angiography
CTD	connective tissue disease
CTLA-4	cytotoxic T-lymphocyte-associated antigen 4
DGI	disseminated gonococcal infection
DILS	diffuse infiltrative lymphocytosis syndrome
DIP	distal interphalangeal
DISH	diffuse idiopathic skeletal hyperostosis
DLCO	diffusing capacity of the lungs for carbon monoxide (diffusing capacity)
DM	dermatomyositis
DMARD	disease-modifying anti-rheumatic drug
dRVVT	dilute Russell viper venom time
dsDNA	double-stranded DNA
DVT	deep vein thrombosis
DXA	dual-energy X-ray absorptiometry
EBV	Epstein-Barr virus
ECG	electrocardiogram
EDTA	ethylenediaminetetraacetic acid
EGPA	eosinophilic granulomatosis with polyangiitis
ELISA	enzyme-linked immunosorbent assay
EMG	electromyographic/electromyography
ENA	extractable nuclear antigen
ESR	erythrocyte sedimentation rate
FABER	flexion, abduction, and external rotation
FDG	^{18}F-fluorodeoxyglucose
FFS	five-factor score
FM	fibromyalgia
FSH	follicle-stimulating hormone
GALS	Gait/Arms/Legs/Spine
GAVE	gastric antral vascular ectasia
GBM	anti-glomerular basement membrane
GC	glucocorticoid
GCA	giant cell arteritis
GI	gastrointestinal
GIOP	glucocorticoid-induced osteoporosis
GPA	granulomatosis with polyangiitis
GU	genitourinary
HAART	highly active anti-retroviral therapy
HIV	human immunodeficiency virus
HLA-B27	human leukocyte antigen B27
HR	hormone therapy
HSP	Henoch-Schönlein purpura
HTLV1	human T-cell lymphotropic virus type 1
HUVS	hypocomplementemic urticarial vasculitis syndrome

ICU	intensive care unit
IF	immunofluorescence
IFA	immunofluorescence assay
IgA	immunoglobulin A
IgG	immunoglobulin G
IgM	immunoglobulin M
IIF	indirect immunofluorescence
IL-6	interleukin -6
IL6R	interleukin 6 receptor
Im Cx	immune complex
INR	international normalized ratio
IP	interphalangeal
IRIS	immune reconstitution inflammatory syndrome
IV	intravenous
JIA	juvenile idiopathic arthritis
KD	Kawasaki disease
LAC	lupus anticoagulant
LFT	liver function test
LD/LDH	lactate dehydrogenase
LH	luteinizing hormone
mAb	monoclonal antibody
MCLN	mucocutaneous lymph node
MCP	metacarpophalangeal
MCTD	mixed connective tissue disease
MPA	microscopic polyangiitis
MPO	myeloperoxidase
MRA	magnetic resonance angiography
MRI	magnetic resonance imaging
MRSA	methicillin-resistant *Staphylococcus aureus*
MS	multiple sclerosis
MSK	musculoskeletal
MSSA	methicillin-sensitive *Staphylococcus aureus*
MTP	metatarsophalangeal
NCS	nerve conduction study
NSAID	nonsteroidal anti-inflammatory drug
OA	osteoarthritis
PA	posterior-anterior
PAN	polyarteritis nodosa
pANCA	perinuclear antineutrophil cytoplasmic antibody
PDE5	phosphodiesterase 5
PET	positron emission tomography
PFT	pulmonary function test
PIP	proximal interphalangeal
PM	polymyositis
PML	progressive multifocal leukoencephalopathy
PMN	polymorphonuclear leukocyte
PMR	polymyalgia rheumatica
po	orally
PR3	proteinase 3

PsA	psoriatic arthritis
PTH	parathyroid hormone
PTT	partial thromboplastin time
q	every
RA	rheumatoid arthritis
RBC	red blood cell
RF	rheumatoid factor
RP	Raynaud phenomenon
SC	subcutaneous
SD	standard deviation
SERM	selective estrogen receptor modulator
SI	sacroiliac
SLE	systemic lupus erythematosus
SLR	straight leg raising
SNRI	serotonin-epinephrine reuptake inhibitor
SpA	spondylarthritis
SRC	scleroderma renal crisis
SSc	systemic sclerosis
ssDNA	single-stranded DNA
SSRI	serotonin reuptake inhibitor
STIR	short tau inversion recovery
SVV	small vessel vasculitis
TA	Takayasu arteritis
TB	tuberculosis
TCA	tricyclic antidepressant
TIA	transient ischemic attack
TMT	tarsometatarsal
TNF	tumour necrosis factor
TSH	thyroid-stimulating hormone
UTI	urinary tract infection
WBC	white blood cell

Contributors

Lori Albert, MD, FRCPC (Editor)
Associate Professor of Medicine
University of Toronto
Staff Rheumatologist
University Health Network, Toronto Western Hospital
Toronto, Ontario

Volodko Bakowsky, MD, FRCPC
Associate Professor of Medicine
Dalhousie University
Division of Rheumatology
QEII Health Sciences Centre
Halifax, Nova Scotia

Michael G. Blackmore, MD, FRCPC
Community Internist and Rheumatologist
Toronto, Ontario

Denis Choquette, MD, FRCPC
Professor of Medicine
University of Montreal
Full-time staff Rheumatologist
Notre-Dame Hospital, CHUM
Institut de Rhumatologie de Montréal
Montréal, Québec

Paul Davis, MB, ChB, FRCP(UK), FRCPC
Professor of Medicine
Division of Rheumatology
University of Alberta
Edmonton, Alberta

Aurore Fifi-Mah, MD, BSc, FRCPC
Clinical Assistant Professor
University of Calgary
Rheumatologist
South Health Campus
Rheumatology Clinic
Calgary, Alberta

Mary-Ann Fitzcharles, MB ChB, MRCP(UK), FRCPC
Associate Professor
Division of Rheumatology
Alan Edwards Pain Management Unit
McGill University Health Centre
Montreal, Quebec

Stephanie Keeling, MD, FRCPC, MSc
Associate Professor
Division of Rheumatology
University of Alberta

Staff Rheumatologist
562 Heritage Medical Research Center
Edmonton, Alberta

Patrick Liang, MD, FRCPC
Associate Professor
Rheumatology Division
Department of Medicine
Université de Sherbrooke
Sherbrooke, Québec

Heather McDonald-Blumer, MD, MSc, FRCPC
Associate Professor of Medicine
University of Toronto
Staff Physician
University Health Network and Mount Sinai Hospital
Division of Rheumatology
Toronto, Ontario

Janet E. Pope, MD, MPH, FRCPC
Professor of Medicine, Division Head Rheumatology
University of Western Ontario
St. Joseph's Health Care
London, Ontario

Éric Rich, MD, FRCPC
Assistant Professor
Director, Rheumatology Program
Université de Montréal
Rheumatologist
Hôpital Notre-Dame du CHUM
Montréal, Québec

David B. Robinson, MD, MSc, FRCPC
Associate Professor of Medicine
Head, Section of Rheumatology
University of Manitoba
Winnipe.g., Manitoba

Kam Shojania, MD, FRCPC
Clinical Professor and Head, Division of Rheumatology
University of British Columbia
Head, Division of Rheumatology
Vancouver General Hospital
Head, Division of Rheumatology
St. Paul's Hospital
UBC Rheumatology Postgraduate Program Director
Vancouver, British Columbia

C. Douglas Smith, MD, FRCPC
Associate Professor and Head
Division of Rheumatology
The Ottawa Hospital and
University of Ottawa, Department of Medicine
Ottawa, Ontario

Muxin (Max) Sun, MD, FRCPC
Fellow, Department of Rheumatology
University of British Columbia
Vancouver, British Columbia

Evelyn Sutton MD, FRCPC
Professor of Medicine and Medical Education
Dalhousie University
Director of Arthritis Center of Nova Scotia
Halifax, Nova Scotia

Regina M. Taylor-Gjevre, MD, MSc, FRCP(C)
Professor of Medicine
Head, Division of Rheumatology
Department of Medicine
Royal University Hospital
University of Saskatchewan
Saskatoon, Saskatchewan

Index